SOUL
SERVCE

Sisters
Good Bless!
Christine Cowgill

SOUL SERVICE

A Hospice Guide to the Emotional
and Spiritual Care for the Dying

Robert Cowgill, MD
Christine Cowgill, MS,CRC

BALBOA.
PRESS
A DIVISION OF HAY HOUSE

Balboa Press books may be ordered through booksellers or by contacting:

Balboa Press
A Division of Hay House
1663 Liberty Drive
Bloomington, IN 47403
www.balboapress.com
1-(877) 407-4847

Because of the dynamic nature of the Internet, any web addresses or links contained in this book may have changed since publication and may no longer be valid. The views expressed in this work are solely those of the author and do not necessarily reflect the views of the publisher, and the publisher hereby disclaims any responsibility for them.

The author of this book does not dispense medical advice or prescribe the use of any technique as a form of treatment for physical, emotional, or medical problems without the advice of a physician, either directly or indirectly. The intent of the author is only to offer information of a general nature to help you in your quest for emotional and spiritual well-being. In the event you use any of the information in this book for yourself, which is your constitutional right, the author and the publisher assume no responsibility for your actions.

Any people depicted in stock imagery provided by Shutterstock are models, and such images are being used for illustrative purposes only.
Certain stock imagery © Shutterstock.

Printed in the United States of America

ISBN: 978-1-4525-6678-8 (sc)
ISBN: 978-1-4525-6679-5 (e)
ISBN: 978-1-4525-6680-1 (hc)

Library of Congress Control Number: 2013900708

Balboa Press rev. date: 01/30/2013

For my late husband, Robert Cowgill. In memory of his pioneering work of service in the hospice area and to his vision of a world where death is embraced as an opportunity for growth amid the challenges it presents.

Helping, fixing and serving represent three different ways of seeing life. When you help, you see life as weak. When you fix, you see life as broken. When you serve, you see life as whole. Fixing and helping may be the work of the ego, and service the work of the soul.

~ Rachel Naomi Remen, MD

Table of Contents

Preface

IN THE PAST, the physician was a medical father figure, accepted into the family. He or she served by being deeply involved emotionally and spiritually with patient care. Routinely treating sick patients in their homes and dispensing empathy and compassion, they were paid with gratitude, love, and acceptance. Their fee was structured so the family could pay what they could afford. The undersupply of physicians ensured a crushing workload, and leisure time was not part of the equation. Although the physician was also attributed a Godlike omniscience—which may not have been earned—based on knowledge and respect, as well as on the emotional connection that was created.

Today everything has changed. The average patient contact is fewer than thirty minutes. There are physicians who practice in large groups with days off, evenings off, and weekends off call, and whose responsibility is limited and narrowly defined, such as heart, kidney or breast specialists. We expect to make comfortable salaries; drive luxury cars; take frequent, expensive vacations; and send our children to the best schools.

Instead of a direct contract between us and our patients, with payment of an agreed-upon fee, we now have the insurance industry brokering every transaction, regulating care, and contributing to inflationary pressures with their own costs. The gratitude, love, and acceptance, which previously contributed significantly to the physician's compensation package, has diminished dramatically.

We may be making more money today, but the personal and job satisfaction costs have been significant.

A complete shift in the concept of service occurred that required virtually all practitioners today to try to keep whatever emotions they may feel toward or about their patients repressed so their reasoning ability is not influenced by them. While our predecessors had only emotional support and empathy in their black bags, we have only our rationality. We are not accepted into anyone's family, we are uncomfortable about having any emotional or spiritual connection with our patients, and we sorely miss the love, acceptance, and esteem we expected to earn as we care for the sick.

When there were few effective interventions to change the natural history of disease, progression and death were accepted consequences of a serious illness. Now that many diseases are considered curable, or at least treatable, the only acceptable outcome is complete cure. The scoreboard is unequivocal: success equals cure, and failure equals death. In the 1970s, cardiopulmonary resuscitation (CPR) was developed to revive the heart after a cardiac arrest. The success rate was sufficient to encourage us to apply this intervention to any hospitalized patient initially, believing everyone deserved the chance to live longer. We residents were paged whenever someone's heart stopped, and we would race into the room with a drug cart and start medications, heart massage, and ventilations to try to "save" a life. No one was allowed to die without this heroic effort to forestall the death.

It did not take long to realize patients with terminal illnesses and a poor quality of life needed to be spared this final assault, and the do not resuscitate (DNR) order was born. The art of medicine often entails dancing in the gray zone between the white light of appropriate aggressive care and the darkness of futile care. While death is still acknowledged to be inevitable, acceptance of it has become more difficult for us because of the promise of medical improvements and breakthroughs. Physicians and patients alike believe we should never give up fighting for a cure, and as a consequence, many of us perish in intensive care units while undergoing active treatments.

The lessening of emotional bonds that characterize today's physician–patient relationships is a major cause of malpractice litigation, and the empathy we used to feel has been replaced by a healthy fear of lawsuits. (The only response that makes sense is to get into a defensive mode and order more tests, consultations, and follow-up exams than you really think are necessary.) Practicing defensive medicine requires being counterintuitive, not listening to your "gut" reactions, repressing your emotions, and acting joylessly from a place of fear. It is not possible to make an accurate diagnosis and proceed with appropriate treatment in a cost-effective manner from a defensive posture, and doing it certainly takes a lot of the fun out of doctoring. No one can guess how much health-care costs would drop, and the quality improve, if the threat of baseless lawsuits disappeared.

Physicians, more than any other professionals, have seen death first hand and dedicated our lives to forestalling it. We are conditioned to look for new treatments and therapies, and we as a group are the least accepting of our own or anyone else's death. We have posed death as the enemy, and we are usually less than graceful when our role shifts to engineering a "good death."

There is no one correct way to die, and each individual has to plot his or her own course. However, Dr. M. Scott Peck articulated the essential elements of a good death in *Denial of the Soul: Spiritual and Medical Perspectives on Euthanasia and Mortality*. It is natural, not a suicide, and should be painless. The dying person has opportunity to heal relationships, move toward forgiveness and reconciliation, and work through the existential suffering inherent in dying toward acceptance. The family and friends have had closure, and there has been time to adjust to the loss gradually.

The physician can be involved in the process of a good death on a high service level. It is possible to create a balance where we can return to the service of compassion and emotional involvement without jeopardizing medical care. This can become the new standard of practice for skilled and compassionate physicians in dealing with distressed terminal patients.

Everyone deserves a good death.

— Robert Cowgill, MD

Acknowledgments

I WOULD LIKE to thank the people I interviewed for this book who allowed me into their professional and private lives. They shared on a deep and personal level their firsthand experiences with end-of-life care. I am especially grateful to those dying patients who allowed me the honor of sharing their last thoughts on their journey home. Their candor allows us to further understand the needs and concerns of those ready to make their final transition. I deeply appreciate the hospice community that supported me in this book project. They allowed me to interview their employees and patients who provide the wisdom that is the foundation of the concept of true soul service.

I am so very grateful to Ruth Donnellan, who assisted in putting me in touch with Dr. Raymond Moody. Dr. Moody has broken barriers and shed much light on the subject of near-death experience as a naturally occurring, cross-cultural, and universal phenomenon. It was my privilege to interview Dr. Moody, who gave so generously of his time, sharing his thoughts and insight into how much more we need to study this still virtually unknown area of life after life and accept the death process as a natural and probably spiritual one.

I am so appreciative of the loving support and assistance of my daughters, Jaclyn Parrish and Jennifer Sugarman. Dan Greenwood was most helpful with his technical assistance. Marlena Freeman was a valuable asset with her research and help in contacting medical and nursing schools.

Last, I am thankful for the constant hard work and research of Elizabeth Ireland. Elizabeth was instrumental in bringing this book project to fruition. It is a project my late husband had envisioned as an embodiment of his life's work, as he strove to change the way we view death and dying in America, as well as develop a better understanding of the need to make every death experience a good one for all concerned.

Introduction

WHILE WE WERE on a weekend vacation with friends, my husband, Robert Cowgill, died unexpectedly of a heart attack. He was sixty-two. It was inconceivable to me that such an active, healthy man could leave this earth so quickly and with no real warning. I so desperately missed not being able to tell my husband of twelve years I loved him and would dearly miss him.

The subject of death and dying, especially in America, is abhorrent to most of us. We simply do not want to think about it until we have to. Almost all hospices require a terminal diagnosis of six months or less. Even then, most actively dying people resist the need for hospice until they are in almost the last few weeks or even days of their lives. Yet, we all die at some point. No one gets out of this life experience physically alive. Last time I checked, the mortality rate was 100 percent. It is not a question of if we are going to die but when. Unless one dies in an accident or from a sudden death, during the last phase of our lives, there is an opportunity to heal ourselves and others, to bring a final sense of peace and closure to our life experience here on earth. Yet, so often those last months or weeks are spent in a futile attempt to deny, put up a brave front, or search for a long-shot cure and not address the inevitable situation at hand.

That scenario is what my late husband referred to as "the train wreck death." Family members often long estranged remain so, or they spend time arguing over treatment instead of just being present for their dying loved one. They do not use those precious final weeks or days to let go of past resentments and simply tell each other they love one another. There is an opportunity, often lost, to use forgiveness to heal ourselves emotionally and spiritually.

After his death, I came across Rob's notes for a book on hospice and end-of-life care he planned to write. As I read through Rob's notes, one section jumped out at me. It was on the different definitions of helping people versus serving people. It read like a really good sermon. I actually felt as though my own consciousness was raised, and I was able to go to work for a long while with more awareness of my own ability to be of service to others. It made me cognizant that so often I was trying with good intentions to "help" people but missed the mark on "serving" them. I knew I had to share this information with others, especially those directly involved in the end-of-life care process. If it made an impact on me, maybe it will speak to the heart spaces of those involved with such care or any person involved in the helping professions.

I contacted and began to interview those wonderful people who are on the front lines, in the trenches so to speak, of end-of-life care about how they saw themselves as being of service. These chaplains, social workers, doctors, and nurses opened up on a very intense personal level, disclosing what was in their hearts in a way that was above and beyond what I would have expected.

Ultimately, death is a personal event. And only those who experience it know the definitive truth about it. Perhaps you are picking up this book because you are a baby boomer, part of that aging population, and perhaps death is in front of you—the death of a loved one, perhaps a parent or spouse, or maybe even you are facing it.

This book will share the evolution of hospice and end-of-life care in this country from the creation of an approach to physically care for the terminally ill to a new philosophy of service at the highest level for those at the end of life. It emphasizes the work of the caregivers—professional and volunteer—who feel it is a privilege to provide a comfortable way station between this world and the next. It also highlights the myriad organizations that have come into existence to relieve the emotional suffering of those at the end of life. It offers choices on how one can approach the final life event: death.

It was an honor to participate in this project, which was so near and dear to my late husband. I hope this book will resonate as truth within the reader and allow us all to act as servants to make the final exit a more peaceful, enriching experience for ourselves and our loved ones.

In service,
Christine Cowgill

Part I

The Patient

*The fruit of silence is prayer; the fruit of prayer is faith,
the fruit of faith is love; the fruit of love is service,
the fruit of service is peace.*

~ Mother Teresa

I believe that imagination is stronger than knowledge—myth is more potent than history—dreams are more powerful than facts—hope always triumphs over experience— laughter is the cure for grief—love is stronger than death.
~ Robert Fulghum

CHAPTER ONE

Evolution of End-of-Life Service

DYING IS A life event. What would our lives and our culture look like if we regarded death as if were starting a new phase of life? It would be much like getting married, having a child, starting a new job, or moving to a new place. Think about the eagerness and excitement (and/or stress) that occurs with each of these movements throughout your life. What if we looked at death as merely another one of these experiences? It was apparent over and over in my research and interviews that death is not the end. It is merely the doorway through which we enter our next life experience.

Death comes to us all in one way or another. In the United States, the 2010 census counted the population at 308,745,538. Of that number, the Centers for Disease Control and Prevention expects the mortality rate to be 838 deaths per 100,000 population, or 2,587,287. The truth is every one of those counted in 2010 will die at some point, including you and me.

In our culture, death has a bad reputation, and we seem to approach it in two ways. The most common way is to simply ignore it, either thinking it is something that is not going to happen to us or that we will think about when the time comes, never knowing how or in what manner that time will come. The not so common choice is to admit it, confront it, accept it, think about it, make choices about who we are, and live our lives in the present so that when the time comes, we are able to minimize the suffering we may experience. Instead of "raging against the dying of the light," as Dylan Thomas encourages us, why not be prepared at the end of life to move "gently into that good night"? No matter what choice you make, it is not possible to avoid the experience. The choice of how you approach death is up to you, but the inevitability of death is beyond your control. Since we only have the opportunity to die once, we should choose to do it well.

Is death the enemy? Many doctors feel so. Trained to fight for life at almost any cost, it is possible for them to feel they have "lost" when a patient succumbs to a disease or condition and death has "won." Death is not considered a natural conclusion of one's life.

Do we deprive people of having a good death? If you can choose, what kind of death do you want? What would you like that experience to be like? So much attention in books, movies, and documentaries is now given to the end-of-life experience, it is possible to think about death in a new light and make choices that affect that experience.

In the sense that death is a reciprocal event, no one dies alone. It has the power to give and receive service at both ends of the spectrum. Those who die reap the benefit of those who care for them; those who care for them reap the benefit and honor of sharing this shattering and illuminating life event with those who experience it.

Think about those in our lives who will help us through that portal into our next existence. Let's take a look at the evolution of end-of-life care—how we look at death—where we have been and where we are today.

THE HOSPICE MOVEMENT

THE WORD "HOSPICE" is common in our society. But sometimes there is confusion over what hospice is, as if it were a particular place where one goes to die. In reality, it is a type of care and a philosophy of care that is available almost everywhere a person lives. It focuses on comfort care, addressing the symptoms of those at the end of life. The hospice philosophy and care were designed to address not only the physical issues that one experiences at the end of life but recognizes many other things are going on as well, including physical, emotional, social, or spiritual symptoms. It can take place as an inpatient facility devoted to hospice care, in a nursing home, through visiting nurse programs in the patient's home, or at an assisted living center.

Today, we are familiar with people who go into hospice or receive hospice care. But it was not always so. In the nineteenth and early twentieth century, people died at home. Eventually a shift occurred and it became an accepted practice for people to die in a hospital setting. Occasionally they still died at home, but most were admitted into a hospital for a serious illness and then remained there until death.

In the past, hospice care was mostly associated with religious orders rather than with the secular medical profession. It has been evolving since the eleventh century, when the Knights Hospitaller of St. John of Jerusalem opened the first hospice in Rhodes. It was meant to provide a refuge for travelers and to care for the ill and dying on a pilgrimage to the Holy

Land. When the religious orders were dispersed, hospice care also ended. In the 1600s, it was revived by the Daughters of Charity of Saint Vincent DePaul in France, and there was a hospice in Dublin, Ireland, started by the Religious Sisters of Charity in the late 1800s. At that time, there was an epidemic of tuberculosis and typhoid, and hospice provided for those afflicted with these diseases. Eventually, the Sisters of Charity expanded internationally.

In the late 1800s in the United States, Rose Hawthorne Lathrop, Nathanial Hawthorne's daughter, was a friend of Emma Lazarus's, whose poem, "The New Colossus" is engraved on the base of the Statue of Liberty. Both women came from wealthy families, and when Emma was dying of cancer, there was plenty of money to provide for her care. However, for the terminally ill poor, it was not uncommon to be banished to Blackwell's Island, a horrible place that included a prison. Rose and Emma shared a mutual seamstress who became ill with cancer and did not have money for care. Rose wanted to help her. So in the fall of 1896, she took a three-month nursing course at New York's Cancer Hospital, moved into a three-room, cold-water flat on New York City's impoverished Lower East Side, and began to nurse the poor with incurable cancer.

Eventually, Alice Huber joined her, and together the expanded, eventually buying property in Westchester and moving into a much bigger facility in New York City. They became cofounders of the Dominican Sisters of Hawthorne, and in 1939, Alice Huber opened a house in Atlanta, which still exists. They are known as the Servants of Relief for Incurable Cancer and provide nursing home services, but only take care of terminally ill cancer patients. Their care is free.

The modern hospice movement is attributed to Dame Cecily Saunders, who, beginning in the 1950s, emphasized focusing on the patient rather than the disease and introduced the notion of "total pain," which included psychological and spiritual as well as physical issues. She was able to share her philosophy through a series of tours of the United States. Eventually she opened St. Christopher's Hospice in London, which has been a model for other hospices and is known worldwide as a pioneering hospice. It continues to do high-quality work with the terminally ill.

Contemporary with Saunders was a Swiss psychiatrist named Elisabeth Kübler-Ross, who made a study of the social responses to terminal illness while living in Chicago with her American physician husband. In 1969, her best seller, *On Death and Dying*, was published and remains a classic today. It had a tremendous influence on how the medical profession began to treat the terminally ill. Almost everyone on the planet is now familiar with Kübler-Ross's five stages of dying—denial, anger, bargaining, depression, and acceptance.

These two women—Saunders and Kübler-Ross—were the pioneers of the modern hospice movement and had a profound impact on the hospice movement as we know it today.

The AIDS Epidemic

THE HOSPICE MOVEMENT, as such, didn't become more commonly known in the United States until the 1990s. As an illustration, in the early 1970s, a friend's father died in the hospital three weeks after he was diagnosed with cancer. There was nowhere else to send him, and treatment at home was not an option. When her mother died many years later, she died at home, part of a new hospice program that provided nursing support and care. Her parents died much differently, her father unaware, not told, "because he couldn't handle it." Her mother knew every step of the way, knew what to expect and had support and the best pain relief medication at the time to support her through it. Her father died at 8 p.m. on a Saturday, while his wife was visiting him. Her mother died at 3 a.m., in her own bed, surrounded by family.

The AIDS epidemic had a tremendous amount to do with change in orientation to hospice. It created the need for a compassionate way to care for young people who comprised a large demographic of those who became infected with a horrible disease and needed precise and caring medical attention. Indeed, it is possible to think in terms of the service all those young men and women provided to the hospice movement. It was through their deaths that the minds and hearts of caregivers across the country were opened to creating caring spaces for them to die.

For example, Clyde Johnson was a CFO for a large hospital in the late 1980s, when he became aware of a considerable discharge problem for his hospital regarding AIDS patients. When the hospital could no longer keep them, where could they go? Their families had often disowned them, and their partners had died. In the beginning, people were even afraid to be in the same room or to even physically touch those afflicted with the disease.

His wife, Metta, is a nurse and relates that when she first started working with patients who were HIV positive, she was employed in the oncology department of a hospital. She would go into the waiting room and immediately know who was new or different. Instead of calling out a name, she would approach the person and ask if he was the new patient. Then she would introduce herself and escort him to the examining room. Sometimes she would touch his arm or shoulder. The patients often asked her if she realized what they had. She would tell them that she was well aware why they were there. Many times she got the response, "But you touched me!" She would simply say, "I think we know how it's contracted." This couple's experiences caused them to combine efforts and create an inpatient hospice where those with HIV could be cared for and treated.

SERVICE

HERE IN THE West, we do not embrace death. We shun it. We do not want to think about it. We would prefer to ignore it, so we are totally unprepared when it happens to us or a loved one. However, it is something that we need to become more conscious of, not in a bad or fearful way—just in knowing our time here is limited. And since that is true, what does that mean to each one of us personally and emotionally? Am I living my passion? Am I doing what I'm supposed to be doing? Can I be more aware? Am I demonstrating love for those I profess to love? How can I be more spiritual in my day-to-day life?

The medical professionals, chaplains, social workers, and volunteers interviewed for this book felt universally that their work was a mission, their life purpose, and that they were lucky to do it. Their orientation was to be of highest service to those dying and to act from the heart space. But it is not only the medical and hospice professionals who serve their patients today. The dying have a very important purpose. By allowing those whose life mission it is to serve the dying, they are served and serve. As one interviewee said, "That's why I feel like, since the nineteen years that I have been with this company, I have grown spiritually, I feel like I'm serving a purpose in life. I feel like this is my mission in life to help serve people." The woman who made this heartfelt comment is not a chaplain; she is a certified nurse's aide, and she feels serving the physical needs of her patients allows her to grow spiritually. She sees it as her mission in life to do the work she does.

That is the ultimate evolution of end-of-life care—to love what you do, feel that you are lucky to be able to do it, and then feel like you make a difference to those you serve.

Throughout the whole of life one must continue to learn how to live,
and what will amaze you even more dear friends,
throughout life one must continue to learn how to die.
~Seneca

CHAPTER TWO

The Patient

THE PATIENT IS the hub in the wheel of the death experience. When a person is in the process of dying, there are dynamics in every single family and with every single person in their community. It is important to be able to bind those dynamics together—children, coworkers, family, friends, neighbors, and pets. Everything needs some clarification on some level. The search for some kind of peace and resolution comes through those connections. It is not uncommon for everything to revolve around the person going through the process. It is almost as if time is suspended. If the experience is family centered, the family priorities shift, and if the person is to die at home, he or she often literally and figuratively becomes the center of the family.

CONNECTION

MOST DYING PEOPLE do not want to be alone. This does not mean they constantly want physical company, but they want to feel connected to those around them, to their loved ones, friends, even the caregivers who see them on a regular basis. To serve that person, it is important for all caregivers to be open to seeing and understanding what he or she might be feeling or thinking and the individual might be behaving in a certain way. It is of value to acknowledge and validate the needs of the person and the process the patient is experiencing. It is through connection that this can happen. There is a need to determine what the dynamics are with the individual patient and his or her family. These dynamics could positively or negatively affect receptivity to the level of care. When you are tuned into the other person and are able to feel the connection between the two of you, it is possible to know what they want and to serve him or her on the highest level. The way to connection is through communication.

COMMUNICATION

WE LEARN THROUGH our ability to communicate. Learning entails more questions. You want to know more, so you ask more. As Dr. M. Scott Peck states in *Denial of the Soul: Spiritual and Medical Perspectives on Euthanasia and Mortality*, (New York: Harmony Books, 1997), 152, "People tend to learn best when they have a deadline."

There does come a point when you know the answer is in the question. That is when the epiphany, or aha moment, occurs. Your knowing is on more than one level. This is possible for the patient and the caregiver. That is the catalyst for change, and you are never able to look at the event, concept, or experience in the same way. Change has happened at a fundamental level.

The urgency of illness is a great opportunity to push through old blockages and talk openly and honestly. However, families are often afraid to bring up anything emotionally challenging. They are concerned that it might cause further pain to the loved one. There is a need to be honest now about what is wanted to communicate— to release old wounds and give and receive forgiveness for hurts, small and large. Sometimes talking about disease changes the anxiety and fear and diminishes loneliness and isolation. For true communication to take place, there is a need to break through those blockages and meet each other on an authentic level.

Prepare yourself to expand your scope of thought. Have you ever had the experience of saying something to someone that was just the thing they needed to hear at precisely the moment? Did you see the look on the person's face? How did it feel? How did it change the relationship? Or did it happen to you? How did it make you feel? That is the power of true connection. Sometimes we only get it in isolated moments and then sometimes we can sit in silence and just be present in that knowing. There is such power in just being present and available to sit with and talk to a person who is dying about whatever he or she wants. Communication can occur on many levels that way.

As Clyde Johnson, puts it,

I would join, usually those guys, out on the front porch of this beautiful one hundred-year old house, sitting on the porch on 14th Street, just being present with the patient. I think that as small as we were we could be family-oriented rather than bureaucratic, like the hospitals and the bigger institutions are required to do. They are not going to ask an LPN or a CFO to go sit out on the porch and be present. So that meant a lot to me, and I think it meant a lot to the caregivers as well. They had that opportunity too. To be present with these terminally ill patients; more so than they could ever be in the hospital, because staffing ratios and things like that kept them away from the bedside. That is a real privilege, too—for people to let you into their personal feelings.

Oftentimes there is a need not to talk about trivial things anymore, but there may be difficulty in expressing that need or having it understood by those who care for them. What is of interest to patients may no longer be the football game, the news, or anything mundane about what is happening to them. Rather, their interest may be on their impact on those around them and what they are leaving behind. One of the ways the professional caregiver can serve the patient and family is to be a catalyst or buffer for the family to initiate those kinds of conversations. Fred Whitehurst, a bereavement manager, said, "You're modeling to them how to be with people when they are taking their last breaths. Have you all told her you love her? People know that now. They are better informed than they have ever been."

How to Talk to a Loved One

FAMILY MEMBERS OFTEN have difficulty speaking with someone who is terminally ill. There is a sense of the "elephant in the room" that no one admits to noticing. Who or what does dying person trust? Use that as a catalyst for conversation or a way to introduce a topic.

In his book *What Dying People Want: Practical Wisdom for the End of Li*fe, (New York: Public Affairs, 2002), 188-192, Dr. David Kuhl makes the point that dying patients do not have unlimited time or energy. It is important to make the best use of the time available, and they want the truth from doctors, family members, and friends. He suggests a number of ways to initiate and maintain a conversation with a loved one.

- Create a private space.
- Eliminate extra noise.
- Make certain both parties are physically comfortable.

- Be aware of your emotions and articulate them. If it is hard for you, say so.
- Explain why it is important to speak to one another.
- Assure the patient that you will end the conversation whenever they want to end it.
- Initiate the conversation; speak clearly and slowly.
- Provide opportunities for the other person to speak. As you listen, suspend judgment.
- Ask questions for clarification.
- Tell the other person how you feel about them.
- If you sense agitation or restlessness, stop.
- Express gratitude.

So often we rush in to do things for our loved ones. However, the best service we can give them may be to hold back, see what they feel they are capable of doing, and allow them to do that. They may soon have to back off of that as well and allow the caregiver to have more and more autonomy over what happens to them.

Meaning

Why me? Why now? These are questions often voiced by those dying. What we understand about ourselves shapes our understanding of time, and time molds our sense of self. What is the meaning of my life; of my death? There is a feeling there must be a reason to have an illness, that it had to happen now, that it is unfolding in this particular way.

Meaning can be discovered through story. It is quite common for dying people to want to share the story of their life, to ensure they had an impact. A study by Harris Interactive in 2005 stated that "a very high percentage of baby boomers considered their real legacy to be the non-financial leave-behinds." In other words, it was the personal stories that reveal not just their family history but also the values, morals, and ethics that the family holds dear. In addition, professional caregivers always remember certain patients who told them stories that affected *their* lives. This is part of the legacy the dying one leaves.

One way to access those stories is through the life review, which is related in another chapter. In addition, dying people may want to write their own eulogy or obituary. Or they may wish to leave a scrapbook or a box with mementos of their life that really meant something to them. Sometimes they will want to go through those mementos and tag them for a particular member of the family. Sometimes, if able, the patient might want to present possessions or mementos to that particular person. This is not to be thought of as some kind of morbid ritual but rather a release for the patient and a way to be able to connect with the person receiving the item.

THE NEED FOR TOUCH

THERE IS A sense of the untouchable when one has a terminal disease. Often, only the medical staff touches the patient—in a professional way—to see if the patient is hot, cold, to check their blood pressure, and so on. Touching and being touched is a two-way street that is an avenue for communication. It is possible with touch to facilitate healing, reduce suffering, and alter pain. You can communicate to the patient that you are there, that you are fully present in that moment. It is another way of being of service, and it is not always necessary to include any verbal communication with it.

Furthermore, Dr. Kuhl states in *What Dying People Want: Practical Wisdom for the End of Life,* (New York: Public Affairs, 2002), 113, "In the nineteenth century and through about 1920, the death rate for babies abandoned to institutions was nearly

100 percent. After 1915 doctors made rules requiring that babies be picked up and carried around several times a day. Handling, carrying, caressing, caregiving, and cuddling became known as basic experiences necessary to the infant's ability to survive."

Touch is essential to everyone, no matter how young or old. When one person touches another, it affects both people. It can communicate your empathy with the person. Franny Singleton, a cancer patient, put it this way: "The empathy is so important, because the patient senses by the touch of somebody if they are just going through the motions or if they really are caring and gentle. I mean, they know. And I know."

Metta Johnson, a director of nursing, said,

It is a very deep joy to sit with someone at the end of their life and touch them. I believe that we can spiritually communicate even when our brains cannot make the words come out of our mouth—nothing verbal going on but I feel like they knew I was there. Sometimes I would just take their arm and rub their arm, and pray peace for them. People just don't understand death very well in this society, and it's possible to pass very peacefully and be a witness to that experience. It affects you very deeply as well and changes you.

Bereavement manager Fred Whitehurst makes a point of touching his patients when he prays with them. "I give them permission just by my behavior. I will go over and touch a patient—you have to be careful with touch—you have to know about pain. But I will touch them as I'm praying, just a light touch. When you have other people that are on the other side of the room, this invites them to come and touch the patient.

SPACE

THERE IS A need to "clear space" to get to what is ultimately important to the person. Clearing of space can be the physical de-cluttering of an area in one's home to make it the space for one to die in comfort and ease. It also can mean clearing emotional space for that person—a sacred space, if you will—to allow that person to be who he or she is and express what the individual needs to say in an atmosphere of love and acceptance.

Chaplain Larry Robert says, "The best dying—dying well— the best experiences I have ever experienced have been when living rooms have been turned into sanctuaries, and that's where the bed is. It's in the middle of the room right when you walk in. The loved one is out of the back room and into the forefront of the family's lives. It's there. I love that so much. When I see that, I know they are doing something right already. That person is always within the mix; they aren't shoved away."

TIME

THERE ARE ALL kinds of time and many metaphors about it. It heals, it works, and it flies. There is time enough, and there is never enough time. Time can be right or wrong. You can take time, lose time, and kill time. It's a gift, a river, a teacher, our father, or as Einstein said, "Time is an illusion."

If you have unfinished business with the people in your life who are important to you, now is the time to address it. When one has difficult personal issues on the agenda, it is easy to put them off to consider later. That later you were thinking about is now. There is no later; there is only now. Especially when faced with a life-limiting timeline, it is best to bring up issues as soon as possible. As motivational speaker Anthony Robbins puts it, "When would *now* be a good time?"

In a way, what Einstein says is especially true for the dying. The dying process comes with its own personal sense of time.

Time is distorted. A dying person might say, "I'm looking forward to my birthday," and at the same time wonder, *Will I be here for my birthday?*

For the dying, the days seem to go by slowly and the weeks quickly. People who are going through the dying process do not plan in the same way as others. Death is "upon one" before they have time to realize it. Time begins to be dependent on the description of what the patient feels is personally most important. There is a sense of being, of existing in a time that does not belong to one. It is a time that extends beyond the limits of one's past and future. At the same time, people with terminal illnesses are capable of amazing feats when they are waiting for a specific family event or celebration in which they wish to participate.

In a friend's case, her mother was dying of cancer when her sister was getting married. While the mother looked forward to the wedding, she would allow no discussion of the wedding being moved up. The date was set, and that was it. On the day of the wedding, she was up, walking and talking with people. For ten hours she participated in the event. When it was over, her health rapidly deteriorated, and in slightly over a month, she died. However, the anticipation of that event was crucial to her, and her need to participate in it was of utmost importance.

It is imperative to *be* absolutely present on every level with a dying loved one. As Fred Whitehurst says, "You are not in a hurry. You don't model as doctors do many times and a lot of the staff, because they are driven by time. You try to change that world."

The last days you spend with your loved ones are memorable ones. You will never forget them. You will carry them with you throughout the rest of your life. As Fred Whitehurst says, "Death changes the world; you know that. You are not the same. We never are. Let's don't pretend like we are going to be."

CHAPTER THREE

Patient Choices

IN END-OF-LIFE CARE today, it is very unusual for the facts of a condition or life-limiting prognosis to be kept from a patient. Instead, there is a tremendous impetus to put patients into the driver's seat of their own care. Each person diagnosed with a serious disease has a personal approach to dealing with the crisis. Most have a positive attitude and are compliant once the treatment plan is decided on. They trust their physicians are competent and knowledgeable, and they expect to be cured, although there is no guarantee. Experience shows that very few patients have had successful outcomes if they have a negative, distrustful, adversarial attitude toward their health-care team or a feeling that they are doomed or deserving of death from their disease.

While the physician is certainly still an essential part of the care plan, the orientation is now more toward how the patient and the physician can work together toward choices and goals. No longer are patients simply told they have to follow a specific plan and to merely trust the decisions the doctor will make on their behalf. The patient does have the ability to meet death on his or her own terms and can make choices every step of the way.

It is possible to express what is wanted, liked, and not liked. In hospice, the goal is to focus on the quality of life, not the length of life. It is important to orient the patient that way as well.

However, that does not mean patients are able to hear that. Patients might know they are not going to get better, but they may not be able to talk to their family about it because of fears and concerns about their family's future without them. The family, on the other hand, is worried about how their loved one is dealing with the prognosis. A large communication gap takes place.

The medical staff is able to take families in that position and walk them all the way through it. Keep them on that track of what their options are and how to compare them to make the best decision. The best medical advice comes when patients are informed and involved.

There is a fundamental choice about death. When a person is faced with the inevitability of death, it is essential to become informed and involved in the process. To a certain extent, death is like the birth experience. It has a significant impact on the family dynamic. It is an event that affects each person differently. There is a window of opportunity where the dying person can model for the rest of the family how to go through the process. This person can be the teacher for the family as they deal with the death of their loved one and help prepare them for the experience of their own death. That is the inherent gift of a gradual death vs. a quick death. Unfinished business can be resolved for the dying person as well as for the members of the extended family.

HOPE

HOPE CHANGES. IT may turn from hoping for a cure, to hoping to feel better or get better, to hoping for closure, to hoping for an easy and peaceful death. Highest service occurs when the staff is able to take that journey with the patient. The patient knows that there is support every step of the way: from the peace and understanding of the progression of their hopes to practical support to keep their fears at bay. Offering hope has to be balanced with the reality of the patient's situation.

Sometimes people do get better. Sometimes it is permanent; sometimes it is only for a while, and they may end up returning to hospice care. Everyone dies, but they often do not do it in the predicted time frame because of the support and help from caregivers. Loneliness and isolation bring death closer. When they are alleviated, there is usually time for things to be done that are important to the client. Providing that opportunity is the highest form of service.

THE DECISION TO USE LIFE-PROLONGING MEDICAL TREATMENT

IS IT IMPORTANT for a patient to fight or to let go? What is important to family members, and how are they dealing with it? The decision really belongs to the patient. Only he or she knows whether it is important to them to fight or let go.

Everyone wants to die with dignity, but what does that mean? For some, just the freedom of choice is paramount. How far does one want to go with life-saving techniques? What does respect for the individual mean to the family and the person who is dying? This means not how far the family wants to go but how far the *patient* wants to go. It is the patient's choice that is paramount. It is the patient's responsibility to put it in writing so that everyone knows it's his or her choice. It's one of the few "controls" a patient has.

To some, aggressive, continuing treatment is worth it, even if it means feeding tubes and experimental drug trials with negative side effects. That person has the right to pursue what can be done to prolong his or her life. Most medical professionals are taught to save lives, and their training, for the most part, is oriented that way. The epiphany for doctors comes when they really see a person experiencing an illness, rather than a patient in some stage of disease process. However, there are doctors who will automatically assume a patient will want to undergo the most aggressive treatments. It is the patient's choice, not theirs. How have you lived your life? Do you really want others to control your death?

However, if one makes an informed decision to choose otherwise, the person has the right to have the best quality of care during the time left. The doctor does not have the right to force radical treatment on someone who is really ready to participate in his or her last life event. It is up to patients to take ownership of their lives, and their wishes should be honored. The family must be considered as well. They need to ask themselves, *If this were me, would I want to be alive if it took all these things to keep me alive? If this were me, what would I like my death to be like? If this were me, am I the type of person I would want around me during this process?*

As much as the diagnosis of a terminal illness marks the end, it also serves as a beginning, an opportunity to ask what the time remaining in your life means to you. *What am I able to do and say in the time and with the energy that remains in my lifetime?*

PARTICIPATION

MOST OF US don't think about death. It's abstract. Even when faced with it, our first response is denial. You cannot die on your own terms unless you choose to be an active participant. Now that sounds a little odd. "I'm going to die anyway, why do I have to act or participate?" It is said that people die the way they live. However, if one has been dissatisfied with life on any level, there is still opportunity for change. It is possible to choose differently.

Anxiety about the effect of a patient's death on the people he or she loves may keep the individual from speaking about that fear or speaking about his or her own fears regarding death. It can create a sense of isolation and aloneness.

Talk with Your Doctor

IT IS RECOMMENDED that the patient have someone accompany them on appointments with their doctor. This person should be someone that can be trusted to take clear and concise notes and not let their emotions get in the way of this important task.

When cancer patient Betty Baker moved to another state to be closer to her sister, she had to change doctors. She was very specific about what she wanted from her doctor, so she interviewed several before she chose one. As she says, "I understood my cancer extremely well, so we could discuss it probably in a lot more detail than he might with another patient. I told him that it was important that he was honest and blunt and straightforward, that I didn't want anything candy coated. So I had that kind of relationship with him, and I think he just felt he could point blank ask was I depressed? Was I moody? Was I having any problems? He would ask me directly; he didn't dance around the issue."

Come prepared for the visit. Bring a written list of questions. Doctors are busy, but they do have time for their patients. If a doctor cannot or will not answer your questions, especially because they want to "save the patient" from worry, consider finding another doctor. The body still belongs to the patient; this is his or her experience. As one cancer patient put it, "This is my life, and I have lived this long without that particular doctor protecting me from myself." People have the right to be involved in their own life, their own illness, and their own death.

Search for and specifically ask for the truth about the prognosis of illness, including the possibility and odds of death. This does not mean a patient has to stop active treatment. It is information. The decision is what to do with that information. Talk about hospice care during this conversation. It will allow the possibility of comfort care to be entertained at an earlier stage in the illness, not just when death is imminent or when all possible medical treatments have been exhausted. Too many times, people only consider hospice care when medical treatments have been exhausted and death is about to overtake them. It is not unusual for people to enter hospice the day they die, because they have neglected to think about it or consider it. Early consideration can lead to a much higher quality of life for a longer period of time.

Hold a Meeting

ONE WAY TO alleviate anxiety is to call a meeting with family and trusted friends to discuss the illness and its prognosis, and to strategize about upcoming issues. The invitation list should include everyone the patient wants to be informed. Duties can be divided up, and suggestions for assistance can be discussed and agreed on.

Worry can often be reduced by introducing certainty. You can create a degree of certainty by developing a plan for care. The meeting should be thought of not in terms of giving up or surrendering, but in terms of planning and creating a way to cover all bases. In preparation for the meeting, one suggestion is to choose a facilitator—other than the patient—who can run the meeting. When everyone has assembled, ask them for their attention, turn off all cell phones, and make sure everyone can stay to the end. It is recommended that a large flip chart be made available so the facilitator can write down everything that is decided.

In the discussion, include the treatment the patient is undergoing, how the patient feels about it, and what the patient wants to do. It is important to be proactive and to ask and answer questions. Topics such as medical information, finances, pet care, and hospitalization or hospice choices can be covered. Chances are the meeting will become emotional, but the goal is to create a community of caring without overburdening anyone who is there to participate. This is also an excellent way to allow people to serve the patient in a way that is truly mutually beneficial.

Making Patient Wishes/Decisions Known

IT IS A wonderful service for the patient and those close to the patient when the patient's wishes are put in writing. It allows loved ones to know what the patient's choices are and gives them permission to take action on the patient's behalf if he or she is unable to do so.

Now is the time to discuss and execute an advanced directive, a living will, a power of attorney, or a DNR order. What kind of care is to be administered or withheld? Does the family know the patient's wishes, and do they understand and agree?

No one can encounter a life-threatening disease with complete equanimity, but patients who feel guilty about their own behavior and participation and who identify exclusively with their bodies have a particularly hard time. A body-centered, materially oriented person has a difficult time in even considering an advanced directive that clearly communicates to the family and health-care team a desire not to have a poor quality life extended by extraordinary measures. This level of acceptance of death can only be achieved by someone who has done the hard soul work inherent in dying.

When she worked in oncology, director of nursing Metta Johnson had a patient she had known for several years. He meant a lot to her, and she knew he wanted to die peacefully. He had a living will and had filled out a DNR order.

Before she left to go out of town, he told her he was ready and prepared to die. While she was gone, he went into crisis while his mother was visiting him, and she insisted the staff resuscitate him. They did, and he spent five more days in intensive care before he finally died.

When Metta returned from her trip, the attending physician told her he was glad she was gone when this happened, as she would have been very upset because the patient's wishes were not honored at all. She later asked the hospital's attorney how the patient's wishes could be disregarded. After all, the patient had had a living will and a DNR order. The attorney explained to her that it is the *living* person who can sue, and the hospital was not willing to take that chance.

Therefore, if decisions have been made and signed regarding directives, make sure they are clear to the family and that the family has agreed to honor them should they be needed. During or at the end of the meeting, copies of the directives can be given to everyone present, so there is no misunderstanding about what is wanted.

When people are diagnosed with a terminal illness, they still have to be considered alive until they are no longer so. There is a period of time when a lot of living can be done and choices made. If you knew you were going to die and there wasn't anything you could do about it, wouldn't you want to live the best way you knew how? Dying well is accepting it, taking advantage of the things the medical profession has to offer, relating to the people around you, and getting as much joy and pleasure out of the things that are still happening.

When we finally know we are dying, and all other sentient beings are dying with us,
we start to have a burning, almost heartbreaking sense
of the fragility and preciousness of each moment and each being,
and from this can grow a deep, clear, limitless compassion for all beings.
~ Sogyal Rinpoche

CHAPTER FOUR

The Fear of Pain and Suffering

WHEN FACED WITH their mortality through a terminal diagnosis, most people are understandably concerned about pain and suffering. They do not want pain; they do not want to suffer physical discomfort through the process. Even with the different levels of pain tolerance people experience, advances in palliative care have made it possible to provide physical comfort.

There is a tendency to think pain and suffering exist only on a purely physical level, but in actuality, pain and suffering have many layers. While they are not mutually exclusive, they are not always the same thing. The experience is much more complex. There can be emotional, psychological, or spiritual components to pain and suffering, and they can be surrounded and infused with fear, anxiety, loneliness, and isolation. Any one of these conditions can make physical pain escalate.

THE GOOD DEATH VERSUS THE TRAIN WRECK DEATH

ALMOST EVERYONE HAS a definition of what a good death is. Overall, most feel a good death is pain-free and peaceful. The patient has everything requested, and family dynamics that can often be quite complex, are in harmony. That is a happy death; the family and the patient are at peace.

The "train wreck death" is a missed opportunity—perhaps emotionally or spiritually—to bring some closure to that life. Old family wounds are left unhealed, or problems or challenges people have had with each other are left unaddressed. Those involved have hung onto their resentments and remained closed to forgiveness. No one is allowed to see how all these things were really not very important after all.

The amount of pain and suffering a person undergoes and how a person deals with it leads directly to the type of death one experiences. Comfort care offers the promise of humanizing the process of dying and focuses medical attention more on improving the quality rather than the quantity of time remaining.

ADDRESSING PHYSICAL ASPECTS

IF PAIN AND suffering were only limited to the physical aspects, it would be comparatively easy to alleviate pain. A relatively new specialty of pain management has been developed in the last few years. Palliative care focuses on preventing, treating, and relieving the pain and other debilitating effects of serious and chronic illness. The methodology employed may run the gamut from traditional Western medicine, utilizing cutting-edge medications, to complimentary care, including such modalities as massage and Eastern medicine. This may encompass everything from acupuncture to chakra alignment. The highest purpose is to control and alleviate the pain for those at the end of life as well as for those who suffer chronic pain. Death may be inevitable, but physical pain is not.

In interviews with professional hospice workers it was overwhelmingly expressed that most patients prefer to die at home, free from pain, and surrounded by their loved ones. Reality is often very different. Many Americans die in hospitals or nursing homes, in pain, and attached to life support machines they may or may not want. This happens despite the medical community's ability to ease most pain and the availability of excellent end-of-life care through hospice and palliative care programs. The percentage of people who opt for hospice only in the last week or even day of life is high. Perhaps this is because of our cultural reticence to discuss death and aging, or because many Americans are not aware of their options for end-of-life care and simply do not ask for them.

Some people are concerned that agreeing to palliative care would mean giving up hope for a cure of their condition. That is not the point of palliative care. In fact, the use of palliative care can help a patient deal with aggressive treatments by alleviating symptoms and controlling pain to assist the patient in his or her fight. According to a study done by the Center for Palliative Care, *The Case for Hospital Palliative Care*, Improving Clinical Outcomes, patients with cancer who receive palliative care were more likely to complete chemotherapy treatment and reported a higher quality of life than those who didn't receive palliative care.

Some patients feel they must make the choice between being conscious and in pain or unconscious and out of pain. Others feel they must "tough it out." It is an individual choice, but if you are in pain, what is your definition of quality of life? Physical pain interrupts everything. It interrupts your thoughts and everything you do, because it prevents you from being able to focus on anything else. If you are short of breath, it is just not possible to focus on anything else. Palliative care helps you achieve quality of life as you define it. It is the job of the palliative care physician to explain the advantages and disadvantages of treatment options so patients can make informed decisions about the management of illness and symptoms and are free to live their life.

When patients have symptoms that are out of control or poorly managed, they may have been experiencing pain for weeks or months. The goal of palliative care is to get pain management to an appropriate level. This allows patients to have better quality time in which they can focus on what is really important to them, versus being wrapped up in a pain cycle.

There are many other benefits to the use of palliative care. Used appropriately, it can complement other therapies. It can be done just about anywhere—hospitals, nursing homes, assisted living facilities, homes, and inpatient hospices. Finally, it can shorten stays in intensive care units and reduce the cost of lab work and other tests. And it is possible to extend someone's life with the use of good palliative care.

According to the American Hospital Association about sixty percent of hospitals have palliative care staff; these are usually hospitals in larger metropolitan areas. If you have received a diagnosis that includes chronic pain or a life-limiting disease, you may wish to seek out a specialist in this area. As always, speak to your primary-care physician about palliative care, but the Internet is a wonderful tool for finding just about everything. Use it to become informed about what is available to you. Be of service to yourself or guide others in this arena to be of service to you by doing the research.

OTHER PHYSICAL AND EMOTIONAL ISSUES

Addiction

BECAUSE PALLIATIVE CARE is a comparatively new medical specialty, concern is often expressed about taking high levels of powerful pain medication, because the patient may become addicted to the medication. Some physicians who are not versed in palliative care worry they will addict patients or even kill them through the administration of too much or inappropriate prescriptive medications. There is also a fear on the part of patients that they will become addicted, and rather than have their pain alleviated to the maximum potential, feel they have to tough it out.

Good palliative care focuses on the pain and its relief. Experts at symptom management and end-of-life care can suggest solutions to the patient, the family, and the physician that dispel some of the myths they may or may not have heard—particularly those associated with certain medications, like morphine. In David Kessler's book, *The Needs of the Dying: A Guide for Bringing Hope, Comfort, and Love to Life's Final Chapter*, (New York: Harper Collins Publishers, 2007), 69, "There is a time to worry about addiction, and a time to make our loved ones comfortable. The two should not be confused." There should never be a need to tough things out.

It is unlikely patients will get addicted to a medication unless they are taking it to have the high. If patients are taking it for physical pain, they are not going to become addicted. It will satisfy the need for comfort. The only choices patients may have to make are in regard to how "foggy" or "drugged" they may feel when taking the medication. Clarity can become an issue. If pain is such that the patient must make a choice between physical comfort and being wide awake for a visit from a grandchild, the pain tolerance level is taken into consideration based on patient choices.

How important is the threat of addiction in the final stages of life? If someone is in the process of dying in a matter of hours, days, weeks, or months and becomes addicted, so what? First, it is the pain that matters and the comfort of that person. Second, should the individual make a miraculous recovery and become addicted, that can be addressed after recovery.

The Double Effect

ACCORDING TO THE Catholic Church, the unintended shortening of a patient's life can be accepted as a potential side effect of treatment, provided the primary purpose of the treatment is to relieve suffering. Underlying it all is the religious and ethical principle called the "double effect," which absolves physicians from responsibility for indirectly contributing to the patient's death, provided they intended purely to alleviate the patient's symptoms.

The *Catechism of the Catholic Church* (New York: Doubleday, 1994), subheading I, Euthanasia, 2279, 608, states:

> Even if death is thought imminent, the ordinary care owed to a sick person cannot be legitimately interrupted. The use of painkillers to alleviate the sufferings of the dying, even at the risk of shortening their days, can be morally in conformity with human dignity if death is not willed as either an end or a means, but only foreseen and tolerated as inevitable.

Physician-Assisted Suicide

THERE HAS BEEN much discussion regarding the ramifications of physician-assisted suicide, particularly for the purpose of alleviating pain and suffering. That discussion rages on. In almost every state, it is illegal. There are rabid proponents on both sides of the issue. Most professional caregivers believe suicide becomes an issue when correct physical pain management has not been done. They believe it is a rare and exceptional case when palliative care is unable to meet the pain level needs.

As M. Scott Peck argues in *Denial of the Soul,* we are here to learn in this lifetime, and facing a terminal illness presents us with the "deadline" most of us need to get the learning done. Depression and emotional distress, coupled with any physical distress a patient might have, serves to stimulate learning and growth. Assisted suicide is illegal. The hospice nurses and social workers interviewed could not recall a single patient who requested it in order to avoid intense suffering. These were professionals who collectively attended thousands of terminally ill patients and saw no need for a change in our current laws on suicide. Life is precious, especially the last few days and weeks of life. And with optimal comfort care, it can be enjoyed and cherished.

Hospice nurses, care technicians, social workers, and chaplains encourage life review, closure with loved ones, and healing of relationships while implementing the medical care plan. They often form a close, loving bond with their patients. Each of us needs assurance that we will not suffer unbearably, and once we have that assurance, we have no need for suicide. That said, it is important to be open to discussing this and any other need patients may have. It can be acknowledged that they have a much greater power to heal themselves emotionally during the death process, rather than a need to hasten death and avoid that healing. There is a sacred obligation to scrupulously consider every aspect of the euthanasia question before we make any changes in our lives.

That aside, there are plenty of books that address this issue, and they are easy to find. Ultimately, like everything else surrounding death, this is a personal issue and choice. However, it should not be considered lightly, and given the litigious nature of our society, it may be very difficult to find a physician to agree to it.

FUTILE CARE

ONE OF THE most inefficient features of our current system is the high cost of dying. There are few reliable signposts for the patient, family, or caregivers to know when further aggressive care is useless. The medico-legal climate seems to force the medical team to err on the side of providing futile care until death intercedes. When this happens, the patient has no opportunity to prepare for death, and the family is likewise forced into having a "positive attitude" until the end, with no hope of closure. It takes skill and courage to make the right decisions at the end of life, and this is true for the patient, family, and friends, as well as the physicians and nurses. Hospice professionals are a valuable resource when questions arise about optimal palliative care and the avoidance of futile aggressive care in preparation for death. The least expensive deaths are often the best, and the most expensive can have devastating, hidden, psycho-spiritual and emotional costs.

ADDRESSING EMOTIONAL ASPECTS

IT IS UP to the medical staff to find a course of action that will alleviate physical pain and suffering. It is up to the patient to find a way to relieve mental and emotional suffering. The truth is no one can assume his or her death will be emotionally painless. However, once physical comfort has been achieved, the patient can move on to the other aspects that are important as the process of dying occurs. The other elements of suffering can include emotional, psychological, or spiritual components. Before someone can truly die free, all these things must come together.

As mentioned previously, people who are dying are still living. It is possible to choose to live every moment left with the highest quality of life available. Palliative care is about living every day you have the best way you can. Part of palliative care is a personal approach that sees the patient as a human being, not just "the colon cancer in room 230."

Restlessness and agitation can indicate suffering that goes beyond physical pain. It may have a more emotional or spiritual base. In the Introduction to Dr. David Kuhl's excellent book, *What Dying People Want: Practical Wisdom for the End of Life*, (New York: Public Affairs, 2002), xvi, Dr. Kuhl tells the story of how he came to understand that suffering is not always physical and cannot always be treated with medication. He had a patient who was dying of lung cancer, and nothing the team did seemed to be able to alleviate her pain. As he describes it,

> With a sense of desperation, I entered her room one more time. Her grimace told me that she was still in terrible pain. I decided to ask a question I had never asked a patient before. Holding Alice's hand, I said, "We haven't been too successful in decreasing your pain. I wonder whether it's possible that the pain in your chest isn't a pain that's coming from the cancer. I have a sense that it is a pain in your heart, one I can't touch." Her eyes told me I had said something that rang true for her. She said, "Yes, the pain is in my heart. It has to do with my daughter, Ruth. She is marrying a man I do not approve of and I told her so. My daughter, my only child, did not want to hear that message. I had to tell her because by the time she realized that he's no good for her, I will no longer be alive. I don't expect ever to be free of this pain, and what's more, unless circumstances change for Ruth, I don't want this pain to be taken away." As we talked, it became clear that she was relieved to finally be speaking with someone about her "real" pain … I knew

that unless the situation changed between her and her daughter, Alice would die suffering the loss of relationship with her only child. There were no medications for the anguish she was feeling.

While it was a relief for Alice to finally share the cause of her pain, her suffering could only be alleviated through an emotional connection with her daughter. Good palliative care is concerned about the patient not just the illness. It can provide emotional and spiritual support and resources, but it cannot resolve a patient's issues for him or her. For that to happen, the patient must release false assumptions and be willing to allow others the space and time to say what they want to say and to do the same. The challenge is to let go of the emotions of the past, the hurts and fears of both parties, and be present for each other.

Through the use of palliative care in hospice, there is a team to serve the patient. This team approach in end-of-life care functions on a high level of service. While medical staff can address medical issues, social workers can address the psycho-social issues, and chaplains can address the spiritual, they actually work in tandem to assist the patient in order to make the dying process as easy and comfortable as possible on every level. This allows them to serve in the highest and best way possible.

OTHER EMOTIONAL ASPECTS

Permission to Leave

WHEN PUSH COMES to shove, people with a terminal illness get to a point when they know they are dying. It is not information that can be kept from anyone going through the process, no matter how well meaning the intention to do so may be. The spiritual connection we feel with the rest of the universe is rocked by the chaos of the dying process, and the trust and dignity of our collective souls is shaken. What is the purpose of our existence in these bodies on this earth? It might be to learn how to give up any semblance of power and control and to dance with equanimity toward our deaths, setting an example for those traveling with us.

Most people in the last stages of dying are afraid to go, not for themselves, but for those they leave behind. This seems to apply regardless of the age of the person going through the experience, whether they are eight or eighty. According to Donna Lewis, a pediatric clinical manager for a hospice, dying children are never concerned about themselves. In fact, it's almost universal with adults and children, because they are always worried about everybody else.

When asked what you say to a dying child, Donna suggests, "You tell them when the time comes, when they are getting closer to death, you tell them it's okay for them to leave. You tell their parents to tell them it's okay to leave, that you will always love them, you will never forget them, and the family will be okay because they will take care of each other. But it's okay to let go."

It is the same for adults. You hold their hand, you hold them in your arms, and you tell them you and everyone else in the family are going to be all right. You give them permission to leave.

Grief

DEATH IS ABOUT loss, and loss is universal. Grief is universal. It is not just the family that grieves the loss. The caregiver also grieves, and it is part of their service to the family. Sally Sutton, a social worker states, "I grieve my patients. I may grieve with the family while they are grieving, or I may do my grief aside. But I grieve all along, because I know that's the healthy thing to do, not to bottle it up. Again, the connections with the family are the blessings to me, and are what keep me going."

Whether it is a parent grieving the loss of a brand-new baby or a sixty-year-old child facing the loss of an eighty-year-old parent, it is the same experience. The focus may be on a life not lived versus having lived a life, but both losses leave a hole. Even if the death has been "a good death," those left feel the loss, and it is still important for them to grieve. Those who have not had the experience of reconciliation and release also must grieve.

As a nurse, Lillian Jeppesen took care of an elderly patient who had been estranged from his son for many years. She called the son several times, trying to get him to at least come and see his father one last time. But for whatever reason, he was adamant about refusing to see his father.

As she tells this story,

After his father died, he came to the funeral, but he just sat in the back of the church. He did not participate in the service, just watched. About a month after his dad died, he came into my office and he was just sobbing. He said, "I'm so sorry I can't go back and undo. I wanted to tell him I loved him, and now I can't do that."

So I said to him, "You can still do that. I'm going to give you some paper and I want you to write a letter to your dad." And I told him that if he liked, I would go with him to the cemetery and leave the letter there. Then he could find some release. And he said he would go home and write it. I was pleased when he came back about two weeks later and asked me to go to the cemetery with him. We went and prayed together, and he deposited his letter and then he began to talk to his dad. And for this young man it was a way of healing. I certainly would have preferred that it had been in person—before his dad died. I know he would have, too, but at least this was one way for him to grieve and begin to be healed.

End? No, the journey doesn't end here. Death is just another path, one that we all must take. The grey rain-curtain of this world rolls back, and all turns to silver glass, and then you see it ... white shores, and beyond, a far green country under a swift sunrise.
~ Gandolf, Lord of the Rings

CHAPTER FIVE

Awareness of Death

THE WHOLE FOCUS of end-of-life care is to provide ways for a dying person to experience as much peace as possible in the transition to whatever is next. We all need companionship, respect, and death with dignity and honor—not defined by the resources available to us but by the humanity offered to us. If available, most of us would choose our physical circumstances to be comfortable to allow for that peace. We would prefer a painless death, whether natural or effected by the use of palliative care. We would hope that we are ready to die, have reached acceptance in some fashion, and said all our good-byes.

Almost everyone is familiar with the five stages outlined in Dr. Elisabeth Kübler Ross's 1969 classic work, *On Death and Dying*. They are denial, anger, bargaining, depression, and acceptance. How one experiences these phases is unique to the individual, and some get stalled in one or another phase and never get to acceptance before death. However, death is a personal experience, and how it unfolds for one person may not be the same for another.

Physical Death

The physical aspect of death is the simplest to explain and understand. The dying person will eventually experience a severe lack of energy or physical weakness. He or she will begin to lose interest or withdraw from others. Usually at this point, the dying person begins to experience excessive fatigue. Most of the time is spent sleeping. At this juncture, it is best just to allow the person to sleep. Hearing is the last sense lost, so it is possible to continue to talk to the person, even if the individual is not responsive.

There will be a complete loss of appetite. In our culture, we feed our loved ones. We center our celebrations on food. Care equals food. However, at the point of death, a person simply does not want to eat. In order to understand this, a caregiver must recall a time when he or she was so sick the thought of food was unbearable. So it is now for the dying person. The body simply can't handle the food, and if it is forced into it, it will come out in one way or another. The body no longer has the energy to absorb or process the food that goes into it. If the person finds comfort with ice chips, Popsicles, or lip balm, use that. Allow the person to communicate what he or she wants or needs.

Nearing Death Awareness

As death approaches, the individual may appear to be mentally confused or disoriented. This is the time when a dying person will refer to "others" in the room or see angels or deceased relatives. They may receive comforting messages. Instead of adding to the confusion, it might be helpful to ask, "What do they look like? What are they saying to you?"

The language used by the dying person becomes very important, because it may be symbolic rather than literal. For example, a person who was a lawyer may refer to the need to "have all the papers in order." A military person may talk about getting ready to "ship out." A mother may talk about the need to make sure the "laundry is done." It is important to listen to the language that is used and then observe the meaning rather than the words. These are all clues that the end of life is coming close.

These types of remarkable experiences are very common as death draws near. Two hospice nurses, Maggie Callanan and Patricia Kelly, refer to this process as nearing death awareness in their book *Final Gifts: Understanding the Special Awareness, Needs, and Communications of the Dying.* These statements, once they are understood, show what the person needs in order to die peacefully. It is not uncommon for those at that stage to predict their time of death. Sometimes they can let go and die only after a certain event or condition takes place; a family wedding or birth of a grandchild. Some things Callanan and Kelly recommend when speaking with the dying is to be honest, but let the dying person lead the way. Be sensitive that they may be unable to focus or absorb what is going on around them or with family members. They may not want to visit as much with loved ones as they did before. It is important not to have your feelings hurt but to understand this may be a necessary part of their preparation for death.

The dying often choose the actual moment of death. It is not uncommon for them to die when loved ones are out of the room—even for a very brief time—in order to spare them. For some, it is easier to let go when they are alone. There is no guilt involved, merely a choice on the part of the dying.

IMPORTANCE OF MEANING

AT THE END of life, many feel their life was meaningless, that there was no real purpose to their life. Meaning is not something you can give to another. However, there are ways to facilitate the understanding of the meaning of life and how their life had meaning, but you cannot give meaning to their lives for them. One way in which you can show someone he or she is cared about is to create a life review for the person. You can do it at any time. This deliberate conversation assists the individual in reviewing the events of his or her life and exploring what personal meaning it has.

THE LIFE REVIEW

WHAT IF YOU took the time to go over and review each moment of your life you can remember? What if you got a notebook and wrote down memories of those events? It is always good to start with "catalytic moments" in your life, times when a specific change occurred that sent you in a particular direction. What are the high moments? How did you feel about them? What happened when you first went to school, met your first friend, and graduated from high school? What about marriage? How did you meet? What was the biggest challenge and biggest joy of your marriage? What was the birth of your child/children like? Did you have any special anniversaries, birthdays, or other celebrations? What happened, why was it significant, and how did you feel about it? Start with the relationship with yourself. What is your earliest memory? How did you feel about it? What can you release? What can you forgive yourself about, and what can you forgive others for?

If a patient has no energy to write, get a recorder and allow him or her to add to it as thoughts occur. This can then be made into mp3 and edited or put onto CDs. If there is time and money, it is possible to hire a personal historian, who will assist in creating the memory and then format the whole thing as a legacy to share with others.

If you are the child, review your perspective with the parent. You may find that you looked at things and felt things very differently. You can use this formula to initiate conversation: I feel (*name the emotion*) because (*state what happened*). Your experiences of an event may be very alike or very different.

Recall the moments of laughter, joy, and celebration. Can you name five good things about yourself that you like? Now name five good things that you like about those closest to you. Tell them what you believe; initiate a conversation about those things. As Socrates said, "The unexamined life is not worth living." Take that opportunity now.

The point is not to dwell on the "negative" moments in life, and beat yourself up about those things, but to let them go and to acknowledge the challenges of life, how you met them, and where you lived in joy. Through this process, the meaning of that person's life will come into focus. Do not be surprised if the topic of forgiveness emerges as a chief concern. Dying people often realize forgiveness is an important aspect of completing unfinished business.

There is often a fear of nothingness, that after this life, you just end. No one can say with absolute surety what happens after death, although many people have beliefs that resonate deeply within them and give them peace regarding the next step. However, dying people look for themes in their lives, often for the first time. They want to identify what they have learned and what they have contributed. Sometimes they are surprised at what they find. If you could give a loved one a single gift before death, a life review would be one of the greatest you could give.

After Death

There is a sense of suspended space after a person dies. It is possible for almost everyone in the room to sense the difference.

It is as if the energy in the room has shifted, changed. After the person has died, it is common for surviving loved ones to still sense the person's presence. Sometimes, as in the case of massage therapist Ruth Donnellan, people feel they are notified of the death of a loved one by the individual himself or herself.

Ruth's father was in an inpatient hospice when he died. One afternoon she was working with a client when she started to hear bells ringing. For some reason, she glanced at the clock and saw it was 2:30. At that moment, the thought of the famous Jimmy Stewart movie *It's a Wonderful Life* popped into her head.

Later, when she received the call about her father, she was told his official time of death was 2:26. She immediately remembered the name of the would-be angel in the movie was Clarence. He told Jimmy Stewart's character that whenever a bell rings, an angel gets its wings. Her father's name was Clarence.

The bereaved often feel the presence of their recently deceased loved ones, who seem to be checking in on them. They may hear words; see their image; smell a familiar aroma, such as a favorite shaving lotion; or merely sense their presence. Such contact with the deceased is not to be feared.

I believe it lies within the realm of possibility that ... almost everyone may eventually come to accept intellectually, even without definite proof, that there is another dimension of existence into which the soul passes at death.
~ Raymond Moody, MD

CHAPTER SIX

The Near-Death Experience

WHAT ACTUALLY HAPPENS to a person going through the death experience? What can you expect to happen during your death process? While there is no precise way of knowing without having the actual experience, clues are available through those who have had a near-death experience. The term "near-death experience" was popularized in the book *Life After Life* by Raymond Moody, which was first published in 1975. Dr. Moody was inspired in his research when, as a student, he read Plato, who not only took the after life question seriously but thought it was *the* most important question of existence,

A near-death experience can be defined as an event experienced by some people who have come extremely close to death. It often occurs when someone is either thought dead or declared dead and "comes back" to life. One researcher, University of Iowa professor Dr. Russell Noyes Jr., studied mountain climbers who almost died in falls. He then extrapolated the information from those experiences to theorize what dying must be like. He found these people seemed to have common experiences that include three distinct phases. He called these phases resistance, life review, and transcendence.

Resistance

WHEN FACED WITH the absolute certainty of sudden death, Dr. Noyes states that a person struggles frantically against both the external danger (falling off the cliff) and a strange longing to surrender to the danger and die. When there seems to be no chance of survival, fear disappears and the person welcomes death.

Before the mood of surrender sets in, some oddly irrelevant thoughts may occur. For example, a good friend related the story of being in an automobile accident when she was a child. She was thrown through the windshield of the car, but she vividly remembers her only concern at the time was what would happen to the new penny loafers she had just gotten.

Life Review

MOST ARE FAMILIAR with the phrase "his life flashed before his eyes." In many near-death experiences, this is a very common experience. Time seems to be suspended, and one's whole life literally passes in review. Events and emotions are focused on, remembered, and reexperienced in what seems like the blink of an eye. Even experiences that have been long forgotten may come to light. The person often feels he or she could have made different choices. The individual may be aware of actions from a different perspective and may now feel differently about those choices.

Transcendence

DR. NOYES REFERS to this phase as "a mystical state of consciousness." This final phase in the experience includes feelings of freedom from space and time limits, submission to the inevitable, total truth, and intense emotionality. A feeling of euphoria comes over the person. If this type of experience occurs, it is important to let the dying person talk about it if he or she chooses to do so.

Dr. Moody's research is in alignment with what Dr. Noyes found. He has spent the better part of his life intrigued by a question that seems nonsensical or unintelligible. To him, the classical difficulty for people is when they look at life after death from a rational point of view. As Dr. Moody points out, "What are you talking about life after death? Death just means the final irreversible cessation of life. So when you say there is life after death, you're saying there is life after the final irreversible cessation of life? That just doesn't compute."

Interviews with people of all ages and from all walks of life and professions have convinced Dr. Moody of one thing. As he stated in his interview:

Let's just set aside the notion of an afterlife for the moment. Let's say there may or may not be—let's set aside that thinking entirely and ask what we can infer as a minimal inference from these NDEs [near-death experiences]. In other words, quite apart from whether there is or isn't life after death, let's just look at these experiences and see what they can tell us minimally. What I would say is that even that minimal thing is mind boggling. And it is. That life is a two phased process—first you run it through from the point of view of the actor or protagonist and then at the end you shift and you look at it the other way from the point of view of the other characters involved—and that to me is just astonishing.

Near-Death Experience

DR. MOODY HAS been able to break down near-death experiences of those he has researched in order to understand the process of dying and to identify specific elements. As summarized in his book, *Life After Life*, these include

- The sound of noise—usually ringing or buzzing.
- Movement through a tunnel or tube.
- Sense of being outside one's own body but still able to observe the physical environment.
- Still have a "body" but different from physical body.
- Strange things happen—awareness of others, relatives, and loved ones who have previously died, or the presence of a loving spirit or being of light.
- A life review in which one is called on to evaluate his or her life and includes the playback of panoramic review of major event.
- Some sense of approaching a barrier or border—that signifies the difference between life and death.
- Told or senses that one must go back; the experience of resistance due to the desire to stay in overwhelming joy in the present.
- Somehow reconnects with the body and returns to consciousness.
- Affects the person who experiences it profoundly.

As Dr. Moody states at the end of his book *Reflections on Life after Life*, (New York: Bantam Books, 1985), 151. "Most people who have had near-death experiences don't seem interested in proving it to other people. One woman psychiatrist who had a near-death experience told me, 'People who have had these experiences *know*. People who haven't should *wait*.'"

Shared-Death Experiences

WHILE THE NEAR-DEATH experience phenomenon is at the very least interesting, the further study Dr. Moody has done into shared-death experiences is fascinating. This experience occurs when a bystander or witness to a person's death has the same kind of experience as during a near-death experience. In this case, however, the person is not experiencing his or her own death but that of the dying person being visited. The bystander often co-lives the dying person's life during the review.

Moody's book *Glimpses of Eternity: Sharing a Loved One's Passage from This Life to the Next*, written with Paul Perry, explains this phenomenon. Dr. Moody was the first to introduce to this concept as a medical student while speaking with one of his faculty members. When her mother went into cardiac arrest and she tried to save her with CPR, she suddenly felt herself lift out of her body and hover in the room with her now-deceased mother. She then appeared to go with her mother into another realm. When they reached a certain point, her mother went on, and she found herself back in her own body.

Dr. Moody didn't discover more of these kinds of cases until the 1980s, and they came from medical professionals working in hospital environments. By the late 1990s, he had heard stories of shared-death experiences from people all over the world.

While these are individual experiences, they seem to have common traits. A summary of what people seem to experience when "traveling" with the deceased includes:

- The bystander senses a change in energy in the room.
- A white mist often rises above the dying person, something like a cloud of steam.
- The room becomes brighter and is filled with white light.

- It is possible to feel light-headed, and the traveler realizes that he has left his body and is now floating above—may even see the room and his own body.
- The bystander sees the person who has "died," and they "hover" together.
- They may travel through their life in memories, and it may have a panoramic quality, much like the near-death experience. However, many scenes are solely part of the "deceased's" life; but the bystander can experience the deceased emotions in viewing these experiences.
- The room itself begins to expand and change shape.
- A tube seems to open in the room and functions like a doorway through which they both move.
- They experience a beautiful landscape, something like a national park, where plants glow from the inside.
- The bystander comes to a boundary and is aware that he can go no further; the deceased moves on, and in a flash, the traveler is back in his body.
- There is a sense that music has been playing in the background during the whole time, unlike anything ever heard, but once he returns to the body, it stops.
- The bystander is left with awareness that the deceased has survived death and is pain-free and well.

If this isn't unusual enough, when there are several people in the room with a dying person, they may all have the same experience. However, it isn't until later, when they begin to talk about it, that they realize this and are able to recall certain aspects of it.

In order to share a death experience with someone, Dr. Moody believes it requires surrender. In his interview he defined surrender as "accept what is happening and give yourself to the person who is dying. Accepting what is can open a person to many possibilities of what can be."

What this means is that the shared death experience is up to individual interpretation. However, there are so many cases of these experiences it is felt there is validity to them. In any case, if there is any comfort for those going through the dying process of their loved one—if any fears have been eased because of the relating of this phenomenon—they have more than served their purpose.

In his interview, Dr. Moody stated that he feels much more education about near-death experiences is needed.

And I do not mean education from an ideological point of view like the parapsychologists want to put on us as they say, "Oh, this is evidence of life after death." That kind of attitude doesn't pay attention to the patient—that kind of attitude pays attention to the parapsychologist's inner needs. They want to be able to say, "Oh, there's life after death." The role of the clinician here is to say to people, "Well, yes, there are these kinds of experiences and they have characteristics A, B, C, and D and they are not connected with mental illness." And to be able to listen to the patient because people want to talk about these things after they have experienced them. The clinician, to me, should be in the role of an educator and a sounding board—but not to put some interpretation on the experience—like—that's life after death or that's brain damage—either one is unwarranted—that's not the clinical role in this—the clinical role is to be supportive to the people and educating the people.

Two Doctors Who Had a Near-Death Experience

In 1999, Wyoming orthopedic surgeon, Dr. Mary Neal, had a life-changing, near-death experience. In her book *To Heaven and Back: A Doctor's Extraordinary Account of Her Death, Heaven, Angels, and Life Again: A True Story,* she tells how, while in a kayak accident, she overturned and was underwater for fourteen minutes. When she realized she was in serious trouble, Dr. Neal asked for divine intervention. According to Dr. Neal, "I felt a pop and it was as if I had finally shaken off my heavy outer layer, freeing my soul. I rose up and out of the river, and when my soul broke through the surface of the water I encountered a group of 15 or 20 souls who greeted me with the most overwhelming joy I had ever experienced or could imagine."

Dr. Neal now has a changed perspective on how she treats her patients. "How I do my work now as a physician has changed. I think I am a better doctor now, in that I try to treat the whole person, not just the injury." What a gift that experience gave Dr. Neal. Her consciousness was raised to better serve others.

In his book *Proof of Heaven*, neurosurgeon Dr. Eben Alexander shares that he contracted a rare form of E. coli meningitis and was in a deep coma for seven days. The neurons of his cortex were completely inactive. As far as Dr. Alexander knows, he is the first person to have a near-death experience while his cortex was completely shut down and while his body lay in a coma.

Most arguments against the idea of near-death experience have been based on the idea the cortex is malfunctioning or operating minimally during the dying process. Dr. Alexander's condition, however, proved this assumption is not correct as his cortex was not working at all.

During the seven days Dr. Alexander lay in a coma, he entered another dimension, the same one described by countless others of near-death experience. In this place, we are more than our bodies. Dr. Alexander, in his experience of life on the other side, encountered glorified, chanting, winged beings that made joyful sounds. He described floating on the wings of a butterfly with a woman, who later turned out to be his dead sister, whom he never met. This woman imparted a three-part message to him, best described as "You are loved and cherished dearly forever. You have nothing to fear. There is nothing you can do wrong."

What a lovely comfort and relief his message to the dying community brings. All is well, and there is nothing you did wrong, there are no regrets, and you are loved unconditionally.

Accept the things to which fate binds you,
and love the people with whom fate brings you together,
but do so with all your heart.
~ Marcus Aurelius

CHAPTER SEVEN

Voices of the Dying

WHAT DO PEOPLE want at the end of life? Perhaps it is not so different from what they want during life. In fact, they are alive and must be considered so. The essence of who a person is does not change just because they are in the dying process. If anything, they become more of what they essentially are. Whatever the center of their life is and has been—church, work, family, and relationships—remains the same.

Those interviewed for this chapter have made peace with where they are on their journey. They were open and honest in sharing their thoughts and feelings, and we are indeed grateful for their time and generosity. Each demonstrated they were in the acceptance stage of the process. However, it was obvious that acceptance manifested in different ways for each person. It was and is an individual perspective.

The people interviewed ranged in time in hospice care from three and a half years to a few months. They all did so because they felt it would increase the quality of life. However, it is rare that people choose hospice early. We all like to be independent, and the decision for hospice is the ultimate procrastination decision. Most people do not want to deal with the fact they are dying until absolutely necessary.

Just like the rest of us, dying people want specific things. They cannot always vocalize what they want, but it generally falls into certain patterns. These patterns can be categorized into aspects that include physical, mental, emotional, and spiritual needs. These are the areas one focuses on in a laser-like way at the end of life. All else seems to fall away or take on a much lower priority. Time is different for these people. Now closer to death, time has slowed. They are in a waiting phase, where the daily concerns of life are less important than the immediate physical, emotional, mental and spiritual needs.

PHYSICAL

OF PARAMOUNT CONCERN to the patients interviewed is pain management. Diagnosed with stage 4 ovarian cancer in 2008, Betty Baker entered hospice care in late 2011. Having exhausted all traditional and acceptable treatments, she was told by her doctors there was essentially nothing else they could do for her. They recommended she consider hospice. She wanted to stay in her home as long as possible and felt early admission into hospice would allow her to do that.

She participated in treatments prior to entering hospice, because she felt it would give her time and quality of life. It allowed her to travel, see people and places that she wanted to visit, and to find acceptance and closure along her path. When her pain level increased to where it could not be managed effectively, she chose to enter hospice early to increase the quality of her life through control of pain. Betty was relieved that she no longer had to call her sister, who lives nearby, at 2 o'clock in the morning if she was in severe pain. She now can call her hospice, and they give her directions on what to use in her emergency pack and then follow up with her. They can take appropriate action should she need it. Previously, she had no other recourse but to have her sister take her to the hospital or call 911. As she put it, "Hospice can do things my regular doctors don't for whatever reason."

The rest of the patients interviewed are in agreement. They all feel there is a tremendous amount of peace available to them because they know their pain is managed appropriately, and their caregivers will not let them be in pain. None of them were concerned with the issue of addiction. The all felt their pain was being managed appropriately, and when and if the pain level progressed, so would their pain management. For those living at home, it gave them confidence to know they had access to advice 24/7. They only had to call hospice, and they would be advised on what to do. Knowing their pain was being taken care of helped reduce concerns over the issue of pain in general.

MENTAL

THERE IS A need at the end of life to make certain everything and everyone left behind is being taken care of according to the person's wishes. This adds greatly to the dying person's peace of mind. Once all decisions have been made, put in writing, and loved ones completely understand what is wanted, a great deal of stress is alleviated for the dying person. Those aspects are put to rest, and the individual can focus on matters more important to him or her.

There are myriad decisions to be made. When—or will—the person enter hospice? What will it look like? Who will provide medical support? How will everyone's life change? Once those decisions have been played out, the person looks to dealing with legal and/or planning issues.

All of the people interviewed had completed their wills and health-care directives, and they had made their wishes known about their funerals. Social workers can be extremely helpful in the hospice program. They can encourage those discussions and facilitate the ways in which the patient wants those directives known. The social worker can also facilitate communication with the patient's family if necessary. There is a need to have these plans understood so that everyone knows what the patient wants well before it becomes an issue.

Willie Martin, who has been in hospice for three and half years, is very clear and open about communicating with his family about his needs and wants. Nothing is being held back. As he said, "I don't feel like they're keeping anything from me, and I'm not keeping anything from them. When the time comes, I just feel I will be satisfied that everything is going to be in order when I leave. All my business and everything I have recorded will be done. My children know what I want."

For Willie and many others, the key component in this process is communication. At first, talking with the family can be difficult. Once a person is in the acceptance stage, it becomes easier for him or her to talk about almost anything. The key thing is if you want to know something, simply ask. Do not assume you know what the person needs or wants. Communicate directly, and ask what the person would prefer. It is as simple as asking, "How do you want me to talk to you?" Then it is possible to be the best friend in the world by providing just that.

For example, Betty feels comfortable talking about almost any topic. Her line in the sand was what she called "crazy cures." People send her articles or e-mails about how she can cure herself by eating two tablespoons of ground asparagus every day and similar claims. She understands they are well meaning, and the reason they send her these things is because they do not want her to die. She tries to be polite, but in reality, she has little patience for it. That is her viewpoint, and it is not unfair to ask her friends to respect it. On the other hand, someone else going through the process may *want* to hear about those types of things.

Another interviewee, Frances Cotrell, experienced a challenging childhood. Growing up the child of sharecroppers, she learned early that she had to do her part in the fields at a young age. When Frances was very young, her mother left her husband, her younger sister, and her for another man. Her father became an itinerant worker, moving them from place to place. Today, diagnosed with a severe heart condition and at the end of her life, Frances wants to write a book about her experiences and leave it for her children and grandchildren. It is a project that allows her to ease her mental anguish, gives her work to do, and helps her feel as if she is passing on information and wisdom to the next generations of her family.

Betty has found mental peace and it sums up what many of those interviewed feel. She lives each day at a time. "My past is my past. My present is my present, and the future is whatever. I don't control it."

EMOTIONAL

THERE ARE A number of ways emotional support can be offered to the patient at end of life. One way is to participate in group support meetings. No one knows better what a patient is going through than someone else having a similar experience. At these meetings, emotional and social support is offered to the patient. It is up to the patient to determine whether this kind of setting would be helpful. Group support systems can be a way to share experiences and come to the recognition that you are not alone in going through this journey. Sharing with and caring about others can be a beneficial experience on other levels as well. Betty was able to share her background in insurance—particularly in the medical arena—and was able to give as well as receive support from her group. In addition, it is possible to find out about experimental drug trials and other information you can take to your doctor and discuss. Finally, she pointed out you just might meet a really good friend.

Another way is to just visit with the person. Frances lives in assisted living and enjoys social things. She particularly likes it when her extended family comes to see her or when there are events at the facility in which she can participate. She loves having visitors and does not like being left alone for extended periods of time. She has a regular volunteer who comes to see her every week, and she looks forward to those visits.

Frances's husband was sick for nine years with Alzheimer's, and she cared for him at home. It was her intention that she be with him when he died. On Thanksgiving Day in 1985, he went into crisis and was taken to the hospital. The doctor decided to admit him, and while she was working on the paperwork, he died alone in a bed in the emergency room. With this on her mind, her greatest fear is that she will die alone. Her life has been surrounded by people—her family, friends, and her work. Many of them were dependent on her. Her family is very supportive and visits her as much as possible, but if days go by and there are no visitors, it is difficult for her.

This is a very common need for many people at end of life. Frances is fortunate to have her family there for her. But there are also organizations such as No One Dies Alone and Eleventh Hour Angels that provide this kind of support as well. If this is important to a patient, there are ways to ensure someone will be there to hold a hand and see him or her through the death experience.

Sometimes people are afraid to say anything because they do not know what to say. It is difficult for them to understand what the patient is going to be comfortable with, so they skirt the issue or even avoid contact with the person. Just because someone is dying does not mean their likes and dislikes disappear.

The bottom line is that it is important for patients to feel cared for and that they mean something to someone. Frances wants to feel loved. For her, that means she won't be alone when she experiences her death. She feels very blessed that she has a family who is trying to see to that need as much as possible.

Most patients do not want to be a burden on their families. They would rather that they just be there for them. Of course, if a crisis ensues, it is important to the patient's well-being to know family is there as needed. Patients need to be reassured that their end of life care needs have been met. They want the peace of mind that their families will cooperate with the end of life care plan.

Crisis is often opportunity. After Betty had her initial surgery, there were major complications. Her sisters took turns caring for her for the six months it took for her to get back on her feet. Her rehab was very difficult, and Betty had the opportunity to see sides of her sisters she would never ever seen had she not allowed them to help her. Betty rediscovered how kind, warm, and thoughtful one of her sisters truly is. Their relationship was not estranged, but they had lived in different parts of the country for so long, seeing each other rarely, that their connection had weakened. Betty's illness gave them both the opportunity to reconnect and on a much deeper level. She looks at it as one of the gifts her cancer has given her. Today they are very close. She feels through the love her sister exhibited for her, and which she allowed herself to receive, her sister really served her on a much higher level. That service was a reciprocal experience.

SPIRITUAL

ALL THE PATIENTS interviewed felt strongly about a spiritual component in their lives that now makes it easier to face the end of their lives. However, they each express it in very different ways. Some are comfortable in their faith and not looking for help in this area. Others feel a particular need to talk about and share their belief system. While they may reach out to others for help, or welcome the time spent with a hospice chaplain, they almost all agree they do not want someone else's spirituality "forced down their throat." They do not want to be "saved" unless that is a necessary component of their belief system. They ask to be allowed to have their spiritual beliefs accepted by those around them.

For Frances, religion has been at the center of her life. Her father and mother were deeply religious; her father led the choir, and her mother played the piano at the church. Her spiritual life began at an early age. A life review is a good way to come to peace with the reasons for the actions a patient took in his or her life on every level. That is another reason Frances is writing her life story. It is a spiritual journey. She needs a way to bring closure into her life. It is important to her to see all the things that happened to her—negative and positive—and to relive the challenges she faced and come to terms with what she did in order to survive. Knowing she did the best she could in her life releases any residual guilt and creates a sense of spiritual peace. Frances also feels uplifted and loved when her family asks if she would like them to pray with her. She would even like others in her assisted living facility to pray with her, but she knows some of them feel that is outside their duties or comfort zone.

Betty, on the other hand, is only interested in praying with people she knows. While she feels that prayer on any level and in any way is good, she is more comfortable when she knows the person is of the same spiritual orientation as she is. "But I am at peace with that. I'm not afraid. I know that I am loved, and I know that I'm loved by God. I feel that love every day."

Willie feels comfortable because he watches religious shows on television, and they keep him company and give him peace. In addition, his church sends a pastor once a month to see him. He knows he has access to the hospice chaplain should he feel the need, but he is more comfortable being with and seeing those with whom he has a relationship. He feels at peace. He is content and does not feel sorry for himself.

All those on the acceptance phase of end of life feel intense gratitude for their lives and the people around them. One of those interviewed plans to write a letter to her family to be read at her funeral. She is already working directly with the minister who will officiate. While she has told her family how much she appreciates everything they have done, she wants everyone else to know as well. Her family doesn't know about it; it is between her and the minister. She plans to make a point of telling them she is grateful for looking at things humorously, how sharing laughter helps her. She feels life is absurd, and dying can be even more so. At the same time, she is grateful for all the things they do for her, from vacuuming the floor to setting up her Christmas tree and then taking it down. She appreciates everything they do for her when she doesn't have the energy to do them herself.

As with everything in life, whatever experience one has at the end of life is based on choice. One of the patients interviewed told a poignant story about one of her sisters, who had died of breast cancer. This sister was continually bitter and angry; she insisted she die at home and with her family personally taking care of her every step of the way. She didn't feel people loved her, which was the furthest thing from the truth. Whatever they did was not enough. Right up to the last three weeks of her life, she would not let hospice in the house. She insisted her daughters do everything for her. She held onto her resentments to the very end. This is difficult for the patient who told the story, because they have the same family and her experience is exactly the opposite of her sister. She just looks at them very differently from how her sister did.

Overall, spirituality is the most deeply felt and personal matter of all the aspects of the death experience. As one of the cancer patients interviewed summed it up, "I'm very blessed. I think that helps with my attitude, because I feel that I am loved. How can you have a bad attitude when people are that good to you?"

Part II

The Caregiver

If you want happiness for an hour, take a nap.
If you want happiness for a day, go fishing.
If you want happiness for a year, inherit a fortune.
If you want happiness for a lifetime, help somebody.
~ Chinese Proverb

We cannot live for ourselves alone. Our lives are connected
by a thousand invisible threads, and along these sympathetic fibers,
our actions run as causes and return to us as results.
~ Herman Melville

CHAPTER EIGHT

Those Who Serve

THERE IS NOTHING as wonderful or as confounding as caring for the physical and emotional needs of someone at the end of life. It requires so much but, at the same time, gives back to the caregiver, for patients not only receive and caregivers not only give.

Caregivers are also witnesses. They witness the life that is unfolding in front of them. They have the opportunity to shine a light on part of a person's life that might have gone unrealized or unacknowledged. Just to be able to recognize the significance of people sharing their lives at this time assists those involved in their care in knowing it is possible to make different choices in their own lives. Ultimately, what a caregiver does is bear witness to the patient's pain and sorrow and remembers the story of his or her passing. Caregivers walk a fine line between being able to give care and getting in the way.

Most of us can understand and empathize about what it is like to be married, to graduate from college, and to have a child. But the ability to offer the empathetic, compassionate part of ourselves to someone who is going through the death experience is not truly understandable until we go through our own death experience. Being available for someone going through the death process is a dress rehearsal for our own death. After all, at some point in our lives we are going to have to deal with it in a very up close and personal way. Caregivers must ask themselves if they are the kind of person they would like to have near me when they die.

It is a high privilege to be allowed into someone's personal feelings. We wear many masks in our society, and being with people when they let their mask down and tell you what they think and feel is a gift. How important is it to have someone you can cry in front of or with?

It will be the patient, not the caregiver, who decides the depth to which he or she is willing to engage and whether the caregiver will be allowed to be engaged in care. The best way to serve anybody, but particularly those at the end of life, is simply to be present with them, to allow them to be who they are. Sometimes this is the highest and best gift you can give to someone.

The Professional Caregiver

Most people who are in end-of-life care receive a team approach from professionals in health care—a doctor, a nurse, a nurse's aide, a social worker, a chaplain—to address their myriad and complex needs. At the first visit or connection, technical details of what the patient and the family can expect from the caregiver—what the professional is going to do, how they are going to do it, and how often will they visit—is often decided. One nurse feels it is her job to guide the family and give them information. However, they are the ones who have to tell her what is happening, because they are the ones always there. Communication is vital, particularly exchanging information on what is working well and going right.

Discussion usually centers on decisions, activities, or food. What does the patient want? What are his or her goals? Decisions need to be made about how those goals are going to be met. How can this all be managed effectively?

The challenge for the professional caregiver is one of balance. It is important to let the patient know he or she matters and that you care about the individual's life—what's happened in the past and what's happening now. At the same time, there is a need to remain professional. Professionalism is necessary, because the caregiver is only going to be in the life of that patient and the life of that family for a very short time. The message may be it is not prudent to get too involved with those they care for; that boundaries must be established. Most caregivers feel they would not be true to themselves if they did that. It takes a special person with a special practice to allow himself or herself to cross those boundaries when needed.

Everyone on the interdisciplinary team gets to know the patient, and the patient gets to know them. They all keep in mind they are there for a reason, and they have to be there and part of the patient's life when needed. But it is not their job to be the friend of the patient or the family. This is sometimes difficult, because either side in the relationship can recognize this person would make a great friend. However, the priority is helping the family through the dying process. They need to depend on other family members, their church, their neighbors, or friends, with the professional stepping in to offer appropriate support and guidance.

The good caregiver still empathizes with the family and shares their concerns for the patient. They understand what is happening to the patient and the effect it has on the family dynamic. Conversation centers around the needs of a dying person, and those discussions often have to do with topics regarding pain management and personal hygiene issues and how the patient feels about them. Closer to death, there may be discussions about the need to no longer feed the patient. It is paramount to be a good listener, to be able to understand the use of silence, to be present. The professional caregiver must ascertain what these needs are and exactly what the patient and family require, because they are different from family to family. Some families have great support systems, and others have very little.

The attentive caregiver is not only a first-rate professional, skilled in creating comfortable physical surroundings, but must also possess a compassionate heart. One professional caregiver refers to this as "medicine of the heart." It is a point where an exchange occurs between the healer and the patient, in which human stories and human natures have been shared. Both parties are enriched by knowing each other. When this happens, it is possible for the caregiver to do more of the right things at the right time for the patient and family.

Needs of the Caregiver

CONSTANT EXPOSURE TO death and dying is disorientating and personally challenging. Therefore, it is important to develop a sense of acceptance so that one does not get carried away by the apparent unfairness of some people's lot. It is also important to release judgment so that you are not influenced by anything you may be told about a person. Sometimes people have a very difficult end-of-life experience; there may be discord, disagreement, or infighting in the family. This is the kind of life they have created. The caregiver can wish and hope things were different, but perhaps the best gift to the family is just to be present without the judgment of how things are *supposed* to look at the end. This allows them the end they have created.

It is the medical director's job to look after the team, to keep track of burnout, to see how the staff's needs can be addressed, and determine what relief work needs to be done. One medical director uses a "sharing stone" to facilitate discussion for the care team. During a meeting, a stone is passed around the group, and each person is invited to speak what is on their heart. This includes everything from changes in the organization to people they had been serving who died; whatever comes up for them. Once everyone is finished speaking, anyone who wishes may express appreciation for the other members on the team. It is a combination of self-expression and acknowledgment.

It is important for any caregiver to use common sense, to exercise, to have fun, and to express their creativity in ways other than through work. And he or she needs to get enough sleep. Caregivers are often at risk of putting themselves last in terms of care, and they must be cognizant of taking enough time for themselves. The best way to avoid compassion fatigue is to have a friend who does the same kind of work who you can talk with who will listen with an understanding heart. It is difficult for other friends, or even your family members, to understand or listen to the challenges and feelings you have in your work with the dying.

Family and Friends

In addition to the health-care professional, family members, friends, and volunteers assist in helping with the needs of the dying person. These run the gamut of addressing physical as well as mental and emotional needs. Once any unnecessary suffering has been resolved, the most precious thing a caregiver has to offer is the quality of his or her presence.

Quite often the family suffers along with the patient. Most want to do the best they can. How do they judge that? Too often that's the point; they judge what they do, criticizing themselves for not doing enough no matter how much they do. They often feel they are not doing the right thing or, after death, that they could have done more.

The best thing the family can do for the patient is to let go of the ego and learn to listen deeply. They should strive to achieve the realization of moments where they can feel very aware of the tremendous privilege of sharing time with people they love who are close to death.

As Maggie Callanan states in her book *Final Journeys: A Practical Guide for Bringing Care and Comfort at the End of Life,* (New York: Bantam Books, 2009), 28, "Dying people do not ask us to analyze, diagnose or solve their problems. They ask us to understand their anguish and be willing to listen and share their journey, good, bad, as far as we can."

People who love one another are capable of doing amazing, incredible things for each other when they feel needed and appreciated. Listening, paying attention to everything, but especially those things that get your attention are skills that need to be developed. Overall, you need to be your authentic self with the dying person, to pay attention and to be cognizant of cues the patient may be ready to talk about deeper things. These may come from the person's silence or nonverbal messages rather than what the patient says.

There is a need for empathy in order to understand what the dying person wants to know or discuss. Allow the patient to take the lead, but if the person wants you to discuss something, be sensitive to that invitation. To acknowledge and validate the loved one is so important at this time. Convey what is in your heart. "I'm so sorry. This must be awful for you." Or, "Can I sit with you for a while, or would you rather be alone?" When dealing with people who face a serious illness, know they are looking at who is around them, what is around them, what they have done, and what they have lost. Once this is understood, it is possible to achieve a high level of honesty and clarity with each other.

Just as with the professional caregiver, the same considerations for personal needs apply to any of the caregivers whether they are family or friends. Do not be afraid to ask for help from other family members and friends. So often people say, "Let me know if I can be of any help." The truth is they really mean it, but they have no idea what kind of help to offer. Step up. Ask them for specifically what you need. Can you go to the store for me? Would you be willing to pick up some prescriptions? Can you walk the dog? Do you have time to sit with my mother while I get my hair done? Most friends and family members are happy to help with this kind of guidance. If you don't know what to offer, these are the simplest kinds of things you can suggest.

There is also a need for respite time for the family caregiver. They may experience burnout, but for them, there is no professional colleague to turn to. Therefore, if there is an inpatient facility associated with the hospice service working with your loved one, ask if they have respite care. If you can arrange a short time or even a weekend away knowing your loved one will be cared for by a compassionate, professional caregiver 24/7, you can have a much needed rest.

Finally, be of service to yourself. There is a need for solace and bereavement for those left after a death in the family. Take advantage of the help offered to you. There are grief support groups available, and you can usually find that resource and others that are available through a discussion with the social worker assigned to your loved one.

HELPING VERSUS SERVING

THERE IS A profound difference between helping and serving. Helping is based on inequality and draws from strength toward weakness. Helping results in debt of the spirit and causes depletion, hence burnout. Helping may leave the person who is the helper with a feeling of self-satisfaction, but the person is working from the attitude of brokenness. This attitude creates a distance between the helper and person being helped. Helping requires mastery and expertise from specialists in their respective areas. Helping is the work of the ego, and the ego likes to judge and feel superior. Helping is viewed as working on curing the person being assisted.

On the other hand, serving is based on equality and draws from wholeness to wholeness, which results in restoring worth to the person on the receiving end. Serving causes renewal and a feeling of gratitude. The service-oriented person works from a place of trust and integrity, which creates a connectedness and willingness to touch the other person's life in a meaningful way. The act of serving requires surrendering to the mystery and awe of the experience, a willingness to be used for the betterment of the situation at hand. Serving is the work of the soul rather than the ego. Service-oriented people see life as an evolving mystery that is rooted in the holy and sacred, and the object is to heal rather than cure the person being assisted.

Most caregivers feel it is a privilege to do the work they do. It is an honor to walk through the door of a dying person's home and be accepted and valued by the family for the contribution they make. For those who serve, the most important thing is to be there and to keep the patient and the family grounded in reality.

Listening is key, and listening to what the patient wants and needs is essential. And listen to what is not being said—read between the lines—and your own belief systems and prejudices aside. Help them achieve what they really want. The gift the caregiver receives is the removal of fear about his or her own death. By working every day with people going through the dying process, caregivers see death; they appreciate the courage they see as other people face it, and they come to know they can do it, too. Caregivers observe and know they have everything they need to have a good death on their own terms.

As Sally Sutton, a social worker, said, "We are there to serve them. Not to impose our beliefs or tell them what we think ought to happen and help them do what we think that they ought to do. So we're there to help them achieve what they want and not to make them do what we want them to do. So professionals really need to put their own stuff aside and be present and listen."

Sally pointed out the essential difference between serving and helping when she said that helping is perhaps to give the family a list of sitters or to tell them where the VA office is located. Serving them is providing what they need to accomplish their goals and then helping them do it; in some cases, doing it for them. To her, if you have belief in a Higher Power, you have that present in your work every day, and you serve in that name, There is no need to change the belief system of anyone else.

RETURN ON INVESTMENT

IT IS DIFFICULT to imagine there is a return on the investment for your time taking care of a dying person. No one goes into caring for the dying for significant financial reward. However, caregivers know that through their action, they make a difference. Every day it puts them in touch with their own mortality, which is a very clarifying experience. They are brought very close to what it means to be a human being. They are called on to do the very best they can every day.

The ultimate gift of caregiving is that it is the fast track to creating a heart connection with another person. The experience can be so rich, so deep, that it profoundly impacts every person who contributes to the care of the dying, no matter what that level of care may be. It is possible to realize the return you get is in the service you give. When you are working from one heart space to another, your most aha moments and spiritual growth occur. Your compassion to relieve suffering in a truly loving way allows you to discover a power within yourself.

Caregivers are privileged to connect with people when they are most vulnerable. Families share with them their thoughts and feelings on a deep level. You are often not privy to that kind of depth with people you have known for years.

Life lessons come from those who are going through the dying process. Those lessons are sometimes profound and uplifting, and sometimes they serve as examples of what we want to avoid in our own lives. In any case, it is impossible not to be altered by the experience. It is not unusual for people who have had family members in hospice to want to give back. They often end up volunteering for work in hospice, because they so appreciate the help they received during the course of their loved one's final time.

Caregivers in their hearts receive a sense of gratification that perhaps they helped just a little bit. Perhaps they made someone's transition a little easier or helped with a conflicting situation within a family. Perhaps they helped soothe the grief of a parent or child, or assisted in helping someone full of blame and anger come to acceptance.

As Vanessa Brown, a certified nurse's aide, put it, "I feel like I'm serving a purpose in life. I'm on a mission. I feel like this is my mission in life to help serve people."

Everybody can be great ... because anybody can serve. You don't have to have a college degree to serve. You don't have to make your subject and verb agree to serve. You only need a heart full of grace. A soul generated by love.
~ Martin Luther King Jr.

CHAPTER NINE

Those Who Are Called

WHO ARE THE people who work in end-of-life care? If you met someone today and the person told you he or she was a doctor, nurse, nurse's aide, social worker, chaplain, or a volunteer who works in hospice, what would your reaction be? In the experience of those who work in hospice, the reaction is almost always one of disbelief and incredulity: "How can you do that, it must be awful!"

For those who are called to serve, and most feel it is a calling, their work is anything but awful. They work from the heart space, and in their work, they find their hearts expand with love and compassion for those they serve—the patient, families, and friends. Almost without exception, they feel it is an honor and a privilege to serve those at the end of life. That receive great joy and satisfaction from their work and simply cannot imagine doing any other type of work. Overall, they feel that through the experiences their careers have afforded them, their own spiritual growth has accelerated.

These people are just like you and me. They have found a position, a career, a calling that gives them satisfaction and joy way beyond the level most people find in their work. But how did this happen? Who are these people, and how do they do it? Following are just a few of the many stories of the ordinary people who perform extraordinary service.

STORIES OF SERVICE

HOSPICE WORK HAS always been a good fit for Sally Sutton, a social worker. She was first exposed to death when she was only four years old and has seen many losses in her family. This allows her a certain comfort level in dealing with death, as well as compassion for those people and their emotions when going through the process. Her personal mission is to help the patient and family get to that place of acceptance by the time the patient dies.

When she walks in the door, she says she feels as if, "I am held in the palm of God's hands." When she does have to face a difficult challenge, she knows she has a colleague she can go to for solace and support. She considers it the biggest blessing she has in coming from corporate to hospice. As she says, "On a daily basis, I get to connect with families, and I am able to help them accomplish something that they want to do, either prior to or in the process of dying. Where they think I'm helping them, I feel like it's a blessing. That makes me ready to go do more. It's their acceptance of what's going on that inspires me."

As a certified nursing aide, Vanessa Brown knows patients will sometimes talk to her when they won't talk to a nurse or even the chaplain who comes to their house. She feels those confidences are a privilege. In the nineteen years she has been with her hospice company, she knows she has grown spiritually, that her work is her mission, and her job is to let her patients know she cares for and is concerned about them. In return, Vanessa gets tremendous satisfaction, because she knows her work is appreciated. "You have to want to serve people, and you have to want to put yourself out there in all ways to help serve them."

It was when Chip Carson, a chaplain, recognized a need in his community—the HIV community—and was given the opportunity to do pastoral care for people affected by HIV that he found his true vocation. When he first walked into a hospital room at a time when 90 percent of the patients were gay white males, he wore his collar and immediately become conscious of a wall going up around the patient. When he introduced himself by name and stated that he was gay and had HIV, the wall crashed down. There was an opening for him to make contact with those patients. He then felt they could serve each other. "I felt that the worst day in hospice or end-of-life care was better than any day I had before that." Now out of hospice due to health issues, he says he misses it every day.

Unhappy with his retirement, Len Dorrien found a place volunteering once a week at a hospice, where he gets much more than he gives. For over four years, he has volunteered to sit with people who are dying and just talk to them about whatever they want to talk about. He refers to his assignments as "my ladies," as most of them are elderly women.

Because he had been in sales and traveled extensively in his career, he has been to most of the places the people he meets lived or visited, and he is able to connect with them through their mutual experiences. Because he had been in military intelligence, Len learned how to interview people and draw them out. He combines these two skills when talking with people, offering them a much-needed social break. "There is a tremendous amount of satisfaction for me realizing that I am helping the family and that I am helping this person during the last stages of their life." He is often privy to information, because he is objective and nonjudgmental; there isn't the baggage conversations with family can often carry. He feels it is his mission to be totally present and is delighted to meet and get to know them.

Leroy John, a licensed practical nurse, has spent his entire nursing career in hospice. When he first got into nursing, he insisted hospice was not his calling. But he needed a job and thought he would get some experience, perhaps for six months, and then move on. But after Leroy saw the level of care hospice gives people, he decided this was his life work; and this happened after only three weeks. He is now in his seventeenth year. He is married to a nurse who tells him she couldn't do what he does. He insists it brings him a lot of joy and much comfort knowing this is his work. He says, "I work in a soul port. It is a soul port, because we are the last people who send you on to the hereafter."

Clyde Johnson relished the opportunity to start a hospice. From a business standpoint, it made sense to provide an alternative to the high-cost hospital setting as well as skilled nursing care and psychosocial and emotional support for those dying in their thirties, which was their demographic. They wanted to do it in a home-like setting, so they renovated two old homes in midtown Atlanta. They kept the charm but supplied these houses with a high-tech medical delivery system.

Part of Clyde's motivation was that there was a need, and they were able to fill it. But it became much more than that for him. He had no idea how much he would get spiritually and emotionally from his work. As CFO of the large hospital, he rarely met the patients. At the hospice, he would sit on the front porch and visit with them, talk to them, and get to know them; they became friends. After their deaths, he would grieve as well. It was life changing for him. He pointed out that half of his and his wife's friends were divorced, but the homosexual relationships seemed to be much stronger. The partners cared for each other, and their bond seemed much stronger. That impressed him to no end. And as it turned out, two of their three children are gay, and his experiences at the hospice helped him be a much more compassionate and understanding parent.

As a volunteer for the Eleventh Hour Angel program, Diana Kirshner is part of an organization that helps prevent patients from dying alone. Sitting with people in the program allowed her to confront her own fear of death. What she found was,

It made me realize completely that just having someone fully present—there in the body—but also in every other way it means to be really present. It makes a huge difference. It fills my heart; it makes me feel valuable, worthwhile; it satisfies my soul. My spiritual path tells me that we are here to share the love and to give the love and to give back what we've been given. So this is my way of being able to give back what I have been given, literally from God.

Donna Lewis, a pediatric clinical manager, has worked with dying children and their families for over fifteen years and feels it is an honor to come into their lives. She believes the families made a choice, guided by their doctors, but an ultimate choice that it was time for someone to help, and she gets to be that person. She attributes her coming to hospice to her daughter, who is special needs child. Her daughter is an inspiration and a teacher to her, and their relationship enables her to work with children who are dying and their families.

People have asked me, "How do you do this?" And I say, I don't know how I do this. I don't know how I sit next to a dying child, but I think I do this because of my daughter and because of my belief system—that she already did her work in heaven;

she came here to get her body and to teach us what we needed to learn. And I believed this before she was born. So I teased her and whispered to her as she was growing, "Save me a place in heaven." I already know her place is guaranteed. So that is why I can go to children and help them, I think. And that's because of my daughter. So even though I never tell anybody that that is what I believe, it is easier for me to take care of a dying child knowing that their work was already complete before they got here.

As a veterinarian who, at a particular point in her life made the decision to pursue chaplaincy, Dr. Delana Taylor McNac is now program manager for the Pet Peace of Mind program of the Banfield Charitable Trust. But it wasn't until she had to opportunity to go to Ground Zero and work there with her church for a few days that she made the decision to pursue hospice work. She worked in hospice for about five years and observed how important pets are to people at the end of life. One particular patient made an impact on her. He was in a nursing home and grieving the separation from and loss of his beloved pet dachshund. When she visited him on the last day of his life, he was lying in bed, talking to no one in particular, and petting an invisible dog.

That experience inspired her to start a program that was eventually adopted and developed into a national program funded by the Banfield Charitable Trust. It is a perfect blending of both of her careers. As she says,

I think that my job now is to be a mediator between two very different worlds. The organizations that support pet-related programs and rescue organization sometimes have distance from the needs of the person. Having walked in both of these worlds of hospice and pet care, I am in the unique position to help someone who is terminally ill and to share with hospices the important role of pets in the midst of all that. I have the opportunity to be the voice for that person and for the pet that ends up in a shelter wondering what happened.

David Frew also works in pet therapy. His journey began when his wife, Stephanie, was diagnosed with a rare form of cancer. While she was in the hospital, therapy dogs were brought onto her floor. That was it for her. As soon as she returned home, they had their dog, Ranger, certified for therapy work.

Before Stephanie died in 2009, she made David promise he would continue her work in pet therapy. He and Ranger now work all over their home city, and videos of "Ranger Frew" at work can be seen on YouTube.

Because of his military background, former navy chaplain Larry Robert now does a lot of work with veterans. The fact that he understands their background training—survival at all odds—allows him to help them with the transition into death and to create a space where they can stop fighting their own death. He believes the key is not to give up but to let go. Former military members often react to the pain and suffering they go through as if they ought to be able to handle it, even though they may be in horrible pain. When he visits people, he feels he brings a sense of peace more than anything else. "I've learned it's the simple and the quiet. How can I be with that person? It only requires one or two words. Sit. Touch. Just be present. It's the hardest thing. Listening. Truly listening."

As the executive director of BayKids, Devora Kanter Kothari helps create movies that are anywhere from five to sixty minutes in length and conceived, written, and directed by seriously ill children. She feels these films are important, because they help the children express meaning for what is important to them. She also offers opportunities for freelancers or those just coming out of film school to make a difference, serve a specific community, and offer a way to celebrate the lives of these children. Their Website, www.baykids.org, offers examples of how these children have used film to create their message and tell a story they want to share. Devora loves her job and could not imagine doing anything else. She looks at what she does as service.

Finally, Ruth Donnellan, a nurse massage therapist,sums it up.

People always say that those who work in hospice are such angels. I'm not an angel. I'm just somebody doing my thing, paying my bills, going to work, but who is passionate about my work. I am all too human.

I see myself as a conductor on a train. When I was an obstetrics nurse, I welcomed the babies and told them that it was going to be a great place, a good adventure, and they would have all these stories and all these wonderful experiences. Now that I am doing hospice, I'm still the conductor. Only now my patients are going back home with all their stories and with all their human experiences. I'm helping them have a comfortable journey back home. That's all. I'm no angel.

My husband died suddenly and then my best friend died. I was a charge nurse on a floor and had two good friends that I worked with, and within a year, both of them died. I went into hospice—I wasn't conscious of it at the time—but I went into hospice for my own healing.

I think a part of me considered death the enemy, because it had taken away so much from me. Now I was going to make sure my patients were as comfortable as possible and make sure their death was as easy as possible, almost as if I was in defiance of death. Now, after all these years, it's okay. We're okay. I don't have any more regrets or anger. There's healing for me, and you know the thing is even Methuselah eventually died. This is only a journey and being born here and living here, that's not the beginning and it's not the end, it's just a piece of the journey.

Hospice healed me. That's why when people say, "You're an angel," I say, "No, I'm not an angel. The angels sent me to hospice."

Spiritual needs and influences intensify as death approaches.
Addressing these needs appropriately is critically important
in the holistic and compassionate care of the dying.
~ Maggie Callanan

CHAPTER TEN

Spiritual Experiences at Death

EVERY DEATH IS a mystical experience on some level. Almost everyone who works in end-of-life care is on the receiving end of experiences they cannot explain. Often, their patients speak of talking to people who have died before them, as if those entities were preparing the way and communicating to them that everything would be all right. Sometimes there is some kind of physical manifestation after a death that cannot be explained in logical terms. Perhaps this is a type of service we provide for each other that never ends. Perhaps those on "the other side" feel compelled to provide this act of service to those in the process of dying in order to convey their continued love and help them prepare for their next step. Perhaps it is part of what we do after our own death to ease the passing of those we love.

THE PRESENCE OF OTHERS

DURING THE LAST three or four days of life, it is common for a patient to "see" and even converse with loved ones who have died before them. The patient doesn't appear to be afraid at all. In fact, the experience may seem to very normal to him or her.

The family, however, will often have a distinctly different reaction. They feel concerned that the patient is "losing it," or they may feel frightened of what they perceive as the unseen. However, this experience is so prevalent, so ordinary, that there is nothing really extraordinary about it. It is almost as if the patient is walking between two worlds—half there and half here. It could easily lead one to believe those who have gone before us are actually helping to facilitate the transition into the nonphysical world.

Regardless of a person's perspective or belief in the afterlife, those experiences can be thought of as a bridge that can carry us safely to whatever is next. It is not unusual when they start talking about someone who has died in the family as if they were right in the room. This is often exhibited as a stare or a look that goes right through the person who is physically there to something beyond, above, or behind them. The patient may be talking to someone no one else can see or sense. These experiences often reduce stress and give a sense of peace, because the event is so clear, so profound, that anyone in the room at the time acknowledges something significant is going on for that person.

There are many examples of those who appear from the other side. The patterns in these stories are similar: a deceased loved one appears in the room and asks the patient to come with them. Usually the patients are the only one who can see these individuals. Sometimes they will even reach out to those they see in the room. And sometimes patients will ask, "Who are all the people in this room?" when it is only the nurse or the aide who is physically present.

Larry Robert, a hospice chaplain, described a patient with AIDS who told him, "'I know this is going to sound crazy but you're the only person I can tell.' He described in detail a visit he had from his deceased grandmother. It made him feel so good that his grandmother was there, and he was no longer afraid of dying."

Vanessa Brown, a nurse's aide, had a patient who felt more comfortable talking with her than with some of the other hospice team members. He had seen and talked to family members who were no longer alive, and he wanted her advice on whether he should go with them or stay. He also wanted to know where God was. Knowing that the man had been an avid golfer, she said, "He's getting that golf course all ready for you. He's at the eighth hole, waiting for you." They both laughed, but she knew it was the answer he was looking for; it made him feel it was all right for him to die.

When a patient was dying from AIDS, the man's life partner told Chip Carson, his chaplain, that the patient said a friend of theirs had come by the previous night. The friend wanted to know if the patient wanted to go out with him. The partner was concerned the patient was losing his mind because, as he told the chaplain, there was no way it could have happened. Their friend was in a nursing home in another state, ravaged by the same disease. When the chaplain stopped by later in the day, the partner said, "I got a call, and that friend I mentioned died last night. He wasn't talking about going out partying; he was talking about going *out* together!"

Another nurse was very excited the first time she was with a patient who told her about those coming to bring him home. She had read about such experiences, and it was very interesting to her. She loved the fact her patient was speaking to his deceased brother John, who was standing at the end of the bed. He described to her what John was wearing: "It's the same shirt that he always wore." The experience was very real for her patient, and it became very real for her. To her now, that is just the way things happen, and she accepts it.

For Donna Lewis, a pediatric clinical manager, it is not uncommon for her young patients to see "others" in the room. Perhaps young children are open to the experience, because at certain ages, children look at the world as a much more magical place than we do as we grow older. She said the team social worker asked one child who was close to death, "Are you having any dreams? What are you dreaming about, are they sweet dreams?" And the child said that his grandfather came to visit and told him that everything was going to be okay. The nurse described another instance where a child told her mother there were angels in the room. The little girl even described her mother's angel as having red hair and standing right behind her. When her mother asked how many angels the little girl saw, she replied, "Hundreds, I see hundreds of angels."

Whenever anyone has those experiences, it seems like it's not long before he or she is okay. There's no fear associated with the experiences. These experiences can bring such peace to the person who has the experience and those who are made privy to it.

Not Quite Ready

Chaplain Larry Robert had an experience with AIDS patient who lived through a near-death experience. At one point, he was so close to death that the nurses hurriedly got his family into the room. Suddenly, he surprised everybody by sitting upright, taking a deep breath, and becoming completely conscious. Then he said, "I need to go home." Everyone in the room told him he couldn't; he needed to stay in hospice, because he couldn't take care of himself.

From that moment, he began to get better, until he was too well for hospice. When the chaplain visited the patient at his home a few months later, he had taken up his old routine of running and jogging. He described to the chaplain his "death" experience and confided that during it, he was conscious of being able to see the spirits of trees and that flowers had living spirits within them. He was able to actually see the spirit within the flower and came recognize that every living thing has a spirit. Back among the "living," he was able to sense that energy or spirit in everything in his everyday life. It changed him in a deep and profound way.

Metta Johnson, as director of nursing, had a similar experience with a patient who died. The attending nurse verified his death and then stepped out of the room to call her and report the death. When the nurse went back into the room, she found the patient alive. When the director arrived at the hospice, she went to see the patient and asked him, "Well, tell me what happened this weekend. Did you really die?" And he said, "I did. I went down this tunnel, and there was this light and then someone said to me, 'Not yet.' So here I am." The patient died three weeks later, when he was ready.

There was a diabetic man who contracted pneumonia and was admitted to the hospital, where he was placed on a ventilator. He survived, and after leaving the hospital, he felt confident enough to share an experience he had with his doctor. "I felt a presence. It was if that presence held out a hand as if weighing something. A decision was being made about whether I was big enough to keep. Like a fisherman looking at a fish and deciding if the fish were big enough to keep. And then the presence took his hand and threw it, like he was going to throw the fish back. I wasn't big enough to keep yet, and so here I am."

Dr. Dwana Bush was pleased her patient had survived the experience, but in addition, it provided them with a language to share based on the experience. For the next three years of his life, he came to decision points about which way to go with his care. And Dr. Bush would ask, "Are you big enough to keep yet?" And the patient would decide on how he felt about whatever decision he needed to make based on his understanding of God or the spirit that helped him to identify what that meant.

EXPERIENCE OF LOVED ONES AFTER THEIR DEATH

To SHARON SCOTT, a social worker, family members who express a connection or sign from their loved one after death is the most enlightening and exciting part of the work she does. When she goes to visit a family member of a deceased patient and imparts to them the regular information about what happens in the grief process, one of the questions she always asks at the end of the visit is, "Have you had any experience of the deceased?" She routinely gets one out of three responses. The first response is very rare—it is negative or in complete denial. She has had that response perhaps only five times in all the years she has been performing social work.

Much more common is that nothing has happened, and the grieving person has been waiting and wants to know *when* it is going to happen. Her feeling is that when we want something like this to happen, it is often very elusive to us. In addition, you can never really know when it is going to happen. Sometimes it can happen immediately after the death or it can happen five years or even twenty years after death. The most common thing that happens is that her clients will look at her in relief and confess that finally, here is somebody that they can tell what has happened, and she won't think they're crazy. And then they tell her the most incredible stories.

Sally Sutton, a social worker, had a personal experience shortly after her mother died. She was living in a two-story townhouse at the time. Downstairs, in the living room, she had an old, family, wicker swing that was hung from the rafters in the living room. It made a creaking sound when someone swung in it. One night Sally was upstairs in her bedroom, sound asleep, and the sound of the creaking swing woke her up. She thought that was unusual, but now wide-awake, she decided to go downstairs and take a look. Sally went into the living room and saw the swing was swinging, but no one was there. Even her cat was gone. No windows or doors were open, so there was no way air could be moving the swing. Suddenly, she smelled the fragrance of her mother's favorite perfume, which was Faberge's Tigress. A sense of peace came over her, and she realized her mother had just stopped by to let her know she was all right.

Finally, nurse Ruth Donnellan tells a story of an experience that stands out vividly in her mind. There is a tendency to think those with Alzheimer's or advanced dementia simply live in their own world and has no idea of what is taking place around them. Ruth had always instinctually rebelled against that idea. She felt these types of patients might indeed know what's going on, but just not in the way we assume the cognitive function of the brain works. She has trained herself over the years to assume nothing.

So whenever she had paperwork to do, Ruth would pick a patient who was nonresponsive, and that's where she would set up and do her paperwork. She would get a small table, bring her charts into the patient's room, and sit next to the person. Then, she would proceed to have a running, one-way conversation with the patient while doing her charting.

One day Ruth picked a particular patient to sit and chat with. After she was all set up next to the woman, she started her conversation. "Wow, you've lived here your whole life. You probably have so many stories. You know, I go to storytelling festivals. If I wasn't a nurse, I think I'd be a professional storyteller. And here you are, and I don't know what your stories are. Well, I'm just going to imagine them. I imagine you went to tea parties when you were younger. Back in the '50s I bet you held tea parties. I can just see you just dressed up, going to meet your friends, having this great social life."

This woman never had any visitors. She had no family left, and she never had any visitors. But after her initial conversation, Ruth made an effort to stop by from time to time to sit with her. She would say, "Okay, I'm ready to have a tea party with you."

The patient never said a word, never opened her eyes; she was in the last stages of dying.

Then one day Ruth was assigned to the patients on the other side of the hall from this woman, and one of her patients was in crisis. She ran down the hall to get the medication she needed and was running back when she happened to glance over at the room of her nonresponsive patient. In the doorway stood a woman in a broad hat and wearing a very pretty dress with large roses on it. She had on short, white gloves and carried a pocketbook over her arm. She looked straight at Ruth, waved, and mouthed the words, "Thank you." Ruth waved back, thinking, *Oh, she finally got a visitor! I'm going to have to go see who this is.*

After she took care of her patient, Ruth went back to the room where she had seen the woman and found the aides were there. The woman had died. The aides had already called the funeral home, and they were straightening up everything.

Ruth was very sad. She said to the aides, "Well, at least she got a visitor before she died. I'm so happy she got a visitor." They looked at her and told her there was no visitor. But Ruth insisted. "Yeah, the lady with the big hat and the dress with the red roses." Then she realized there was no visitor. It had been her nonresponsive patient. Ruth knew at that moment the woman was there, because she had not been looking for that experience. But her patient had stopped to say good-bye to her, and it was the last thing she was looking for on a busy, busy day.

Part III

Service from the Heart Space

Teach this triple truth to all:
A generous heart, kind speech,
and a life of service and compassion
are the things which renew humanity.
~ Gautama Buddha

Many things are too large to submit to any single adequate definition: love, death, prayer, consciousness, light, and so on. I do not believe it an accident that all such things have some connection to God, the largest, most indefinable and mysterious thing of all.
~ M. Scott Peck, MD

CHAPTER ELEVEN

Recognition of Spirit

DEATH IS A spiritual journey that brings our whole being into question. As hospice nurse Maggie Callanan states in her work *Final Journeys: A Practical Guide for Bringing Care and Comfort at the End of Life*, (New York: Bantam Books, 2009), 145, "When someone we love is dying, all of our feelings, spiritual beliefs and cultural expectations about death become emotionally charged and intensified."

The word "spirit" or "spirituality" has just about as many meanings as there are people. What we each mean and know by that phrase is a different thing. We cannot presume to know what God means to an individual person. We can only know the pull is there, drawing that person to their spiritual home.

You can call the impetus behind spirituality whatever you want: Buddha, God, Allah, the All, the Source, the Universe, the Supreme Being, the Field, the Force. However, at its very core, it all comes down to the same thing—whatever religion or spiritual practice guides one to worship, it is all one, it is all the same, and it is intimate and deeply personal.

As bereavement manager Fred Whitehurst says,

In a traditional Catholic family, being able to have a priest come and do the Sacrament of the Sick can give a patient a sense of completion. Or perhaps a Jewish person can have their rabbi visit them, or an imam can come. Those visits can mean a lot to a family. But it is still not the mystical connection. Perhaps part of the good death is that you have taken care of things here and been true to your faith—your tradition. And some people talk from the spirit, and they don't really need to see their minister. They are simply glad to have some people share with them and listen to them.

Against the backdrop of infinity, our purpose can be made clear. If we are here to serve each other at the highest level, isn't death one of the great teachers? We serve by our example of not how we die but how we live until we die.

IMPORTANCE OF SPIRITUALITY

THE AUTHORS BELIEVE if you put on blinders and say that you will only be interested in the body—you will ignore the spirituality, the emotions, and the mind—then you are robbing yourself of all a physician can do for you.

A dying person feels the need for connection to something bigger than himself or herself. A person's orientation to the spirit can be expressed in a multitude of ways, including religious traditions, a love for nature, connections to family, art, music, or some other way that is deeply personal. Regardless of spiritual orientation, patients often struggle with such questions as "Why me?" or "What will happen to me?" or "What has my life meant?"

These are inherently issues of the spirit. The dying person becomes more concerned about what is in the heart than what is in the head and needs to express personal beliefs, concerns, and fears on that level.

As Dr. M. Scott Peck states so succinctly in his book *Denial of the Soul: Spiritual and Medical Perspectives on Euthanasia and Mortality*, (New York: Harmony Books, 1997), 152, "Dying can be the opportunity of a lifetime for learning and soul development."

However, now is not the time to "save" anybody based on anyone else's religious preferences. Instead, find out what is important to that person and how the individual views his or her spiritual life. Then do what is available and achievable along those desires.

PATHWAY TO THE SPIRIT

SPIRITUALITY IS AN expression of how people relate to a larger whole—something greater than themselves—and how they find meaning amid their suffering. Both the patient and the caregiver can benefit from increasing spiritual awareness. The following references provide a roadmap to raising spiritual consciousness.

Dr. David Kessler worked closely with Dr. Elisabeth Kübler Ross, and in his work *The Needs of the Dying: A Guide for Bringing Hope, Comfort, and Love to Life's Final Chapter*, he suggests five stages of spiritual reconciliation.

Expression

THIS IS ALL about expressing our feelings, no matter how ugly or beautiful they are. If you are not able to talk about it, or it is difficult for you to talk, try writing it down. Keep a journal or simply write a letter to your disease and tell it exactly what you think and feel about it. This was first suggested in Marianne

Williamson's book *A Return to Love,* and it helped many people begin to deal with what is going on inside of them and about what has happened to them.

Responsibility

THIS TIME IT really is all about the patient. Now is the time to face the life-limiting illness head-on. Now is the opportunity for us to take responsibility for everything that happened in our lives. However, there is still a choice about how we can accept that responsibility. If we haven't been the heroes of our life, now is the time to choose to let go of victimhood and choose responsibility. Now is the time to give up what has been done to us and what we have allowed to happen. We have the responsibility to tell our caregivers and/or family members what we really do need and want. We cannot assume they know what we need. If we do, we can plan on being disappointed. It is our responsibility to communicate with them.

Forgiveness

WHAT DOES FORGIVENESS mean? One thing it doesn't mean is condoning bad behavior. We simply release ourselves from the cords that bind us of hurts received or the perception of hurts received. We must recognize that after death, one side of whatever quarrel or disagreement existed is now gone.

There is a famous story about a Hindu man whose son was murdered by Muslims during the religious riots in India in the 1940s. He could not find it in his heart to forgive. He went to Gandhi and asked him, "How can I possible forgive the Muslims? How can I ever find peace again with so much hate in my heart for those who have killed my only son?" Gandhi suggested that the man adopt an orphaned Muslim boy and raise him as his own.

Remember, this is your death. How do you want to die? What things have you done right in your life? Can you expand that now into forgiveness on every level? If you can't do it, ask for help from the higher power, if you believe in one, and counseling if that is available to you.

Acceptance

IT IS COMMONLY thought that to accept something means that we feel it is somehow good or even desirable. The truth is we do not have to like what we accept.

Death is much bigger than we are. Every life is complete. Every person who has been born and died has had a complete life, no matter how short or long it may have been. There is a bigger picture, a cosmic picture if you will, and to cry and complain against the unfairness of what we did or did not have, did not get to do, or whatever is failure to see that picture. As cancer survivor Franny Singleton puts it, "I am going to die no matter what. If you believe in eternity—always has been and always will be—a year or two doesn't make much difference. If you die at twenty or fifty, or even one hundred, if you're looking at time as never ending, it's nothing, you know."

Gratitude

AFTER THE OTHER steps, the person can now be grateful for his or her life—good, bad, and in between.

Larry Robert explains that in his fifteen years as a hospice chaplain, the force of gratitude for life he sees in his patients transcends other experiences. "I find a lot, especially when I was working the HIV community, they would say to me, 'Larry, I'm dying, but this is the greatest gift, because I've been able to realize who I fully am. This disease has brought me to a point spiritually to realize who I am, and I'm okay.'"

His patients finally realized it was not the disease, and it was not the body. They realized they were a spirit and were finally in touch with that.

Finally, there is a Hawaiian spiritual practice called *Ho'oponopono,* which is a form of connection. Basically, the term means "to make right," especially with the people with whom you have relationships. In the Hawaiian tradition, it is thought to be important to align and clean up any past problems in relationships, especially with relatives.

The process instructs you to visualize a particular person you would like to be at peace with. Then imagine an infinite source of love and healing flowing from a source above the top of your head (or your Higher Self). Open the top of your head, and let the source of love and healing flow down inside your body. Let it fill up the body and overflow out your heart and out to heal the person you are thinking about. While this occurs, think of these four phrases: I'm sorry. Please forgive me. I love you. Thank you.

After you finish, you should feel a certain level of peace. If the opportunity to meet and discuss the process with the person you visualized becomes available, you may want to take advantage of that.

FAITH

FAITH IS NOT so much about sets of ideas we are required to follow, but about ways of being that may involve a degree of surrender on some level. Faith does not imply giving up or rejection of self, but the realization there is something more than the physical. People with no spiritual connection often have a difficult time when faced with death, because their fear can overwhelm them. So if one can surrender, let go, and leave things to divine order, or in the hands of God, it will open a space for participating with others on a higher level in the life that is left to be lived.

Faith also allows for boundaries between people to crumble and the recognition of importance and priority in the moment. With faith, listening takes place in a realm of pure relationship, and connection is possible at a much deeper level. Ultimately, death is about trust from a spiritual viewpoint. Trust that there is something coming that is beyond the physical existence. Trust that the next level of existence will be for our highest good.

BEAUTY AND TRANSFORMATION

CHAPLAIN ROBERT BELIEVES there is a sense of beauty that can be achieved for both the patient and caregiver at the end of life. People want to make sense of the life they have lived, to see the patterns, and to acknowledge the spiritual yearning and connect with it. Often they get to a point where no matter what they have done or who they were, they are beautiful now. Their life was beautiful. They have an appearance of the transcendent, almost as if they were getting lighter, were lighter.

It is often at night, or when patients are alone, that the big questions about their beliefs come to the forefront. As Myrna Bond, a director of nursing, says, "It's up to God to do it. He may use somebody that just visits for a day to say something encouraging. We don't try to interpret someone else's experience."

Former hospice chaplain Chip Carson had an experience that perfectly illustrates that concept. He tells a wonderful story of connection between a father and son that was facilitated not so much by who Chip was or what he did, but how he was with a patient.

He went to visit a patient with HIV, and the last time he saw him, the patient's father was with him. The father sat in the far right of the room, against a wall, just about as far way from the patient as he could get. Chip walked into the room, around the bed, and leaned over and gave the patient a big hug. Then, intentionally, he told the patient he had other visits to make but would stop by before he left. Later, when he returned, the father had moved up and was sitting next to his son, holding his hand.

Bereavement manager Fred Whitehurst had a patient who never spoke with anyone. The nurses told Fred he was the only person who came to see the man. Fred hadn't known that. One day Fred had a meeting, so he just stopped to check in, and it looked like the patient was sleeping. So he quietly asked, "Do you want me to leave you alone, or do you want some company?"

The patient opened his eyes, looked up, and said, "Company!" Fred's whole agenda went out the window. The man had never acknowledged his presence before. He was alone and didn't want to be. And because Fred understood that, on that afternoon, he made a difference for that person.

Knowing you have a finite amount of time left can be a gift, an opportunity to focus. How do I see myself living in that time? What is important to me; what falls away? Who do I need to make amends with? If I am in a place of total love, am I connecting enough with others? Social worker Sally Sutton puts it this way.

The patient knows what they want. They know if they are ready to go. Sometimes the spiritual basis is a factor. I have a patient and every time I see her she says, "I don't know why I'm still here. I hope the next time you come, I'm not. I know I'm here for a reason. I don't know why God's keeping me. I'm ready to go—I'm ready to go be with my husband." She believes in God, she trusts in God, she knows He is keeping her here for a reason;

she just doesn't know why—and she's ready. I think most people know before the families know and are ready to accept.

Since Dr. Eben Alexander's near-death experience, he has made a study of quantum mechanics and how it relates to consciousness. As he puts it,

I see science and spirituality going forward, together— science and spirituality as being one, and complementing each other beautifully. Both the religious side and the science side will have to let go of some of the more simplistic dogmatic assumptions and statements, but then science and spirituality and this deeper knowledge of the profound nature of our individual consciousness can move forward, the world will be an enormously better place when we do that.

Ideally we would have access to holistic generalists who have an extensive knowledge of disease prevention and treatment of illness. If necessary, specialists would be readily available to manage more complicated problems. Other practitioners such as massage therapist, acupuncturists, fitness coaches, and physical therapists would assist in maintaining our wellness.

~ Robert Cowgill, MD

CHAPTER TWELVE

Complementary Care

PART OF THE comfort care approach to treating patients at the end of life is to offer complementary services that can be an adjunct to conventional and traditional medicine. The goal of these services is to focus on the patient's quality of life, personal meaning, and alleviation of symptoms rather than on prolonging life or treating the disease.

There are many ways to treat physical pain. What truly makes someone comfortable is an individual choice. While efforts are often, and justifiably, directed toward palliative care, a new breed of therapists, social workers, and other personnel involved in end-of-life care are also incorporating elements of mind and spirit in work with patients who have been diagnosed with terminal illnesses.

The benefits of using complementary care are that they are not invasive and can be done in conjunction with medical treatments a patient already receives. There are many services, tools, and modalities that encompass complementary care. What follows is an overview of some of the ways in which a dying patient's end of life can be enhanced through the use of these different modalities.

THE MIND/EMOTIONAL MODALITIES

THE ARTS CAN bridge inner experience to the outer world of words. Creative arts therapies promote an interactive approach to wellness. The emphasis is on helping individuals take an active part in their healing process and develop outlets for creative expression.

Art

ART THERAPY IS based on the notion that people project their internal world, both consciously and unconsciously, into visual forms. Feelings or thoughts that may be difficult for people to express in words often come more easily with images. It can awaken that language of images, symbols, and metaphors that speak for the deepest aspect of the person going through the dying process. Through movement, poetry, psychodrama, ritual, artwork, and creative writing, a bridge can be built between the inner experience and the outer world of words that can transform what is in the unconscious into conscious reality.

One of the keys to their effectiveness is that the arts provide a nonthreatening opportunity to express feelings that are often too painful for words. The art forms provide a safe structure to uncover, contain, and assimilate the feelings that surface in therapy. Clients and therapists alike find a therapeutic environment that supports creative activity, expressive interaction, physical vitality, and spontaneity can be a growth-promoting and enlivening place to be.

This new direction toward creativity, as well as the newly rediscovered respect for the role art plays in communication and emotional release, is extended to the dying as well as families during the bereavement process as well.

Music

Music therapy began when singers and musicians would come to hospitals to visit patients wounded in World War II. There are several ways music can be of help. The conscious use of music as an adjunct support service is a good example of how the multidisciplinary approach to hospice care seeks to address the total person and his or her family.

Research provides support for music therapy to increase quality of life, alleviate spiritual suffering, provide pain management, and promote relaxation in end-of-life care. Therese Schroeder-Sheker developed a field called music thanatology through the Chalice of Repose Project, an organization that provides musicians to play for people at end of life.

The term "thanatology" is derived from *thanatos,* the Greek term for death. The term "music thanatology" often refers to a specific way of using live harp music at the bedside of dying patients. Music thanatologists view their work as a compassionate, spiritual, and contemplative practice. In hospices and hospital facilities that provide musical support, a family can arrange for a bedside visit by one or two specially trained musicians to sing or play live music for someone who is dying. The purpose of such a music vigil is to provide comfort and support both to the person who is dying and to loved ones.

Pet Therapy

Sometimes friends and family don't know what to say. They may even stay away, not because they don't care, but because they simply do not know what to do or say. They often feel helpless or useless. Pets, however, are always there and are completely nonjudgmental. Pet therapy programs bring animals into the nursing home, assisted living, or inpatient hospice facilities. This type of program usually consists of volunteer owners and pets that are trained to orient themselves to the patients.

Patients will often put up walls and boundaries when faced with a terminal illness. Animals can have almost a magical, calming effect on people. Often when a pet is there—a dog or a cat—and the patient is petting it, the individual is able to relax and begin to talk about what is on his or her mind. It is then possible to really begin to learn about the patient's real needs. Pets do not care what you look like or how you feel, and it is possible for the patient to experience unconditional love when the pet is there.

There are national and local programs that provide support to the terminally ill. Once such is the Happy Tails Pets program, which works in hospice and home-care facilities. An adjunct to many pet therapy programs is the Pet Peace of Mind Program.

Pet Peace of Mind Program

THE PET PEACE of Mind (PPOM) is a national program funded by the Banfield Charitable Trust. It is designed to help nonprofit hospices keep patients and their pets together during the end-of-life journey. The program also helps hospices find adoptive homes for pets, giving patients peace of mind that their pets will always have loving homes. Currently, there are over forty nonprofit hospices across the country that offer the Pet Peace of Mind Program. In this way, patients are able to release worry about what will happen to their pets after they are no longer able to care for them.

Lillian Jepperson, a hospice nurse, was inspired to start a Pet Peace of Mind program at her hospice by a patient who was in an inpatient facility. When he was very close to death, she asked him if there was anything she could do for him. He wanted to go home; he wanted to see his wife and children. Now she knew he had no children. So he shared with her that he had a German shepherd and a sheltie. He just wanted to get home to see them one last time. Lillian felt compelled to see what she could do to help him. When she talked with his doctor, she was told it would be all right as long as she could get a hospital bed and the equipment he needed, and arrange appropriate transfer. She managed it all in a very few hours, because she knew it was very important for him to get home and say his final good-byes to those he loved the most.

As she says, "This program is part of the spiritual and emotional support system for the patient. I would like to see it become a standard in hospice care and not just a program that distinguishes hospices from their competitors or is necessarily what a cutting-edge hospice adopts because they want to do a deeper level of care. I would like to see it be a standard of care where pets are considered part of the family by every hospice, where we take into account pets and their importance in the family."

BODYWORK MODALITIES

Acupuncture

ACCORDING TO RUTH Lever Kidson's book, *Acupuncture for Everyone: What It Is, Why It Works, and How It Can Help You*, (Rochester: Healing Arts Press, 2000), 2, "Acupuncture uses a single therapy—the insertion of needles into the skin—to treat a variety of ailments. Accupuncture can treat all ailments in the same way because it sees them as stemming from the same cause— a disruption of the energy flow or vital force of the body."

Chiropractic

IT IS THE goal of the chiropractic to normalize the relationship between the structure of the body and its ability to heal itself. It focuses on the body's structure—mainly the spine—and its functioning. Although different chiropractors use a variety of treatment approaches, they primarily perform adjustments, or manipulations, to the spine or other parts of the body.

Clarity Breathwork

CLARITY BREATHWORK USES the ancient practice of circular, connected breathing that has been used in cultures around the world for thousands of years, for healing and attaining higher states of consciousness.

Proponents believe that the breath is the connection between the emotional, physical and spiritual components of a person's being. By deepening the patient's own breathing patterns, the technique offers the patient the opportunity to release stress and tension as well as heal and resolve trauma. Clarity Breathwork is described as a safe and effective method to support the ability of the patient to access their own internal healing energy and greater knowing. Practitioners believe that from this place, it is possible to experience a shift in personal understanding and awareness. By breathing fully and consciously, the patient learns to release what he or she has been holding back and to open to the possibility of expanded consciousness, including greater forgiveness and self-love.

Massage

THE BASIC MECHANISM through which massage therapy helps the dying is touch. People who are sick or elderly may be touched very little, especially if their family is not near or their spouse has died, or if they live in a caretaker environment such as a nursing home. These people especially need caring people around them to hold their hand, rub their back, brush their hair, or to hold them when they need someone.

Because of the direct contact massage therapy offers, it provides a way for the dying to relax, thereby reducing the anxiety associated with the process they may be going through.

Massage also provides stimulation, helping residents communicate physically. The reason touch is so powerful is based on the recognition that tactile experiences are the first sensations that greet us at birth. They are also the last perceptions to leave us when we die.

Touch can penetrate the semi-comatose state produced by painkillers and give the person some sense of human contact. In some patients, massage may reduce the request for drugs when it is a part of their treatment routine.

ENERGY WORK MODALITIES

Healing Touch

HEALING TOUCH IS an energy therapy in which practitioners consciously use their hands in a heart-centered and intentional way to support and facilitate physical, emotional, mental, and spiritual health. It is based on the research that there is a magnetic field around the body, and that field can be activated or manipulated to create health and healing.

Healing Touch uses the gift of touch to influence the human energy system, specifically the energy field that surrounds the body and the energy centers that control the flow from the energy field to the physical body. These noninvasive techniques employ the hands to clear, energize, and balance the human and environmental energy fields, thus affecting physical, mental, emotional, and spiritual health. It is based on a heart-centered, caring relationship in which the practitioner and client come together energetically to facilitate the client's health and healing.

Reiki

THE WORD "REIKI" is composed of two Japanese words: *rei*, which means "God's wisdom" or the "Spirit," and *ki*, which is "life force energy." So Reiki is actually "Spirit guided, life force energy."

Reiki treats the whole person—body, emotions, mind, and spirit—creating many beneficial effects that include relaxation and feelings of peace, security, and well-being.

Reiki is a simple, natural, and safe method that everyone can use. It also works in conjunction with all other medical or therapeutic techniques to relieve side effects and promote recovery.

Reflexology

REFLEXOLOGY DEALS WITH the principle that there are reflex areas in the feet and hands that correspond to all of the glands, organs, and other parts of the body. Stimulating these reflexes properly can help many health problems in a natural way and act as a type of preventive maintenance. It should not be confused with massage.

Practiced by the Egyptian culture as early as 2330 BC, reflexology as we know it today was first researched and developed by Eunice Ingham, the pioneer of this field, who published her first book on the subject in 1938.

As with any medical treatment, there can be risks with complementary therapies. It is suggested that if you or a loved one is considering any of these modalities that you select a practitioner with care. Be sure to find out about their training and experience before you engage their services. In addition, make sure you tell your primary health-care providers about any complementary practices you use. It is important to have a full picture of what is being done to manage illness. The end result is safe and coordinated care.

PERSONAL HISTORIES

AFTER SPENDING TEN years as an investigative journalist and untold hours interviewing people for newspaper stories, Massachusetts journalist Kitty Axelson-Berry decided to interview her own mother. She wanted to investigate her own past. The experience was so personally rewarding that the next year she founded the Association of Personal Historians (APH), a trade association for the few writers then engaged in helping the nonfamous put their memories on paper.

A personal historian can help a dying patient leave a legacy for generations to come. The patient is usually provided with a list of questions and then interviews are held. The responses are formulated into a book presentation and range from just the questions and answer to a professionally completed personal biography of everything the person wants included. Copies can be printed and made available to whomever the patient wants to have them.

END-OF-LIFE PARTIES

OF GROWING POPULARITY is the end-of-life party, which occurs before the death of a loved one. End-of-life parties can take the place of, or be used to complement, the more traditional funeral. These parties are designed to allow the dying person to participate in saying good-bye to friends and family. This can be a very healing experience for all concerned. It need not be a big, expensive affair. It can be held in a home, an assisted living facility, or a hospital, with some refreshments and a sharing of stories and memories about the dying person's life. Pictures of the dying person throughout his or her life can be on display, and old home movies could be shared. It can be a wonderful opportunity to tell one another about the special part each played in the loved one's life.

End of life parties do not have to be a formally planned event. Sometimes using a holiday as an excuse for a life celebration can give the same benefit. Lillian Jeppesen, a hospice nurse, relates this story.

Several years ago, I had a patient who had pancreatic cancer, and the first part of October he asked me if he would be here for Christmas. I told him that from his signs and symptoms and the progression of his disease process, I doubted if he would still be here for Christmas. However, only God knows this answer. He laughed and said, "I see." Three days later, when I went to see him again, he opened the door and said, "You were wrong. Merry Christmas!"

As I entered their home, I saw they had a lovely Christmas tree, brightly lit up, gifts under the tree, a beautiful nativity set, Christmas music playing, and his wife was baking his favorite Christmas cookies. The house smelled and sounded like Christmas! He shared that his children, his brother, and sister were coming the following weekend from out of town to celebrate Christmas together. This was a special holiday for them, and the entire family was truly blessed by this event. This patient died on October 31. So it is always important to know of any special wishes a patient may have and try to honor them.

LIFE LEGACY BOXES

LIFE LEGACY BOXES is a nonprofit program formed by Dr. Dwana Bush, who runs a family medical practice and is also certified in hospice care. The project was designed to help patients in hospice care find comfort in the small treasure of their lives.

As Dr. Bush explains,

The whole idea is that there are people that build beautiful things with wood, and they have so much heart, and there are organizations of woodworkers. In addition, many take up woodworking when they are older in life. What we want to do is to match the creative capacity to build boxes with the need that hospice patients have that their life mattered. The boxes are given at no charge, the patient is supported and their life acknowledged. They put whatever they want into the box that has meaning to them and to be passed on to those who survive them; sometimes it is the family that picks and chooses those items to be placed in the box and kept, perhaps handed down generation to generation.

There are also organizations and practices that contribute to the comfort of a dying person merely through their presence.

ELEVENTH HOUR ANGELS

ELEVENTH HOUR ANGELS is a volunteer program that trains people to sit with the dying during the last phase of their life. The program is based on a book written by Barbara Karnes titled *Eleventh Hour Angels*. Usually you go weekly and volunteer for time slots to be present with a patient so they are not alone.

Sometimes it is difficult for families to be present during the death of a loved one. They feel they cannot handle the experience and make a conscious choice not to be present. It is really rather sad; it leaves the patient alone, literally, with whoever is available.

As Lin Tatum, an Eleventh Hour Angel volunteer puts it, "The whole concept is no one dies alone. That's where Eleventh Hour Angels come in. Sometimes there are other family members who aren't in the room. At this point, there is nothing medical left to do; you are just waiting. So we sit with the family or just the patient, and we wait. We sing to them; we talk to them. We always tell them exactly what we are going to do, such as when we are going to put a cool cloth on their head. We are there just to let them know someone cares."

The Twilight Brigade

The Twilight Brigade is similar to the Eleventh Hour Angel program, but it is dedicated to being at the bedside of America's veterans. It is one of the largest end-of-life care communities, and it is their mission to raise society's consciousness about the needs of the dying, especially veterans. They utilize community and professional education, advocacy, and direct service to the terminally ill and their loved ones, ensuring no one need die alone.

Complementary Care Websites

Art Therapy
American Art Therapy Association
www.arttherapy.org/aboutart.htm

Music Therapy
American Music Therapy Association
www.musictherapy.org

Center for Music Therapy in End of Life Care
www.hospicemusictherapy.org

Chalice of Repose Project
http://chaliceofrepose.org

Massage Therapy
American Massage Therapy Association
www.amtamassage.org

Healing Touch
Healing Touch International
www.healingtouchinternational.org

Reiki
The International Center for Reiki Training
www.reiki.org

National Institutes of Health
nccam.nih.gov/health/reiki

Reflexology
International Institute of Reflexology
www.reflexology-usa.net

National Certification Commission for Acupuncture and Oriental Medicine
www.nccaom.org

National Center for Complementary and Alternative Medicine
nccam.nih.gov

Life Legacy Boxes
www.lifelegacybox.org

Association of Personal Historians
www.personalhistorians.org

The Twilight Brigade
www.thetwilightbrigade.com

Too often we underestimate the power of a touch, a smile, a kind word,
a listening ear, an honest compliment, or the smallest act of caring,
all of which have the potential to turn a life around.
~ Dr. Felice Leonardo Buscaglia

CHAPTER THIRTEEN

Training/Orientation for the Medical Professional

As RESEARCH WAS done for the book, it came to light that few medical and nursing schools offer coursework to our upcoming doctors and nurses on the aspects of death and dying. For the most part, when they do, these courses are optional. And here is the conundrum—death is not optional for their future patients; 100 percent of them will, at some point, die. What should medical schools do to address this issue?

Part of the discussion rests in the medical training that insists on seeing death as the enemy that needs to be fought at all costs. How does one "manage" death from this point of orientation? While there can be an appreciation for a course in pain management—and there have been great strides in the development of palliative care programs in schools—should it remain optional? Another part of the problem is there is no one-size-fits-all approach to end-of-life issues. Those that arise in intensive care, emergency medicine, obstetrics and perinatal medicine, pediatrics, and the care of persons with AIDS are individual and do not exactly fit into the oncology model. Physicians should be adequately trained to care for dying persons in a variety of settings.

Back in 1997, Harvard Pilgrim Health Care, Inc., organized a two-day National Consensus Conference on Medical Education for Care Near the End of Life. In a report prepared by Kelsey Meneham, *Rx: More Training Urged for Physicians Treating Dying Patients,* for the Robert Wood Johnson Foundation, (http:// pweb1.rwjf.org/reports/grr/029360s.htm), the eighty-five medical professionals attending the conference recommended that:

- Care at the end of life should be taught as a core professional task throughout the continuum of medical education.
- In all phases of training, students should be exposed to dying patients and to interdisciplinary teams of clinicians and other healthcare professionals who can teach and model the humanistic functions of medicine and who are skilled in palliative care.
- Although the preclinical years have an important role in teaching about end-of-life issues, undergraduate educators should also focus training in the clinical years where key attitudes and life-long practice patterns are learned.
- To succeed in improving end-of-life care, medical schools must train and hire more educators to provide and demonstrate state-of-the-art palliative care. These educators are needed to serve as teachers and role models for medical students, residents, fellows, medical school faculty, and physicians-in-practice.
- Teaching end-of life care to physicians should focus on four major goals: developing appropriate communication skills; acquiring essential technical knowledge for treating

symptoms and relieving pain; learning to address the psychosocial, cultural, and spiritual needs of patients and their families; and developing the ability to reflect on personal attitudes about this work.

We could find little evidence that much progress has been made in implementing these recommendations.

As part of the research for this book, 122 medical schools and thirty-four of the top fifty nursing schools were contacted to determine if they had mandatory courses on death and dying from a psychological, emotional, or spiritual perspective. Also explored was the course offering on palliative care. Only eight schools had these courses as mandatory, and only sixteen had elective classes in those areas. There is a need for mandatory training in our medical and nursing schools.

Physicians are trained to treat diseases. They address a patient to find out what is wrong and then do their best to fix it. Their skills have been honed to care for patients by treating a person's underlying disease, rather than by addressing the complex, often idiosyncratic elements of their suffering. Personal anguish is not part of their medical vocabulary. They are not without heart but without understanding. Today there is a shortage of doctors who truly understand, connect with, and serve those who are at the end of life from an orientation of heart-centered service.

The old paradigm where the healer buttons up "self" regarding psychosocial/emotional aspects of patient care for fear that emotions could "cloud" reasoning needs to change. Under that paradigm, the healer would limit himself to wanting to deal purely in the physical realm. The new paradigm sees illness as four components—spiritual, mental, emotional, and physical—with empathy required to sort out the jumbled and conflicting messages.

Hospice doctor Dwana Bush believes it comes from an impetus of why a person is in medicine to begin with. She says,

Here's my thought—and I used to tell med students this—I encourage anybody in the healing professions— you have to decide do you want to be a health technician or a healing practitioner? The health technician can be very good; they could be a great surgeon or an orthopedist or, you know, have certain skills, but the patients are looking for heart, and so the health technician may be able to give a service—and that could be needed. You have to decide do I have that healing practitioner's spirit—and how does that speak and serve? The other thing I tell students is to look for people who love their work, enjoy their life, and laugh a lot—it doesn't matter what field they are in so much as you let them influence your life. So being around people of good heart, seeing what they do that works, how they handle when things don't work, how they take care of themselves are probably more important than some of the formal techniques and training, because they will be able to form an authentic connection and develop their own creative approaches.

"One of the biggest hurdles to overcome is convincing current and future physicians that dying and death is not a medical failure," says Mary Meyer, who coordinates education projects for Choice in Dying. Her organization is currently working with a group of medical schools that want to develop mentors and standards for teaching these issues. "This is an extraordinary bias to overcome," she says.

Harvard Medical School has developed a preclinical course for medical students called "Living with a Life-Threatening

Illness," which annually enrolls up to 30 percent of the first-year students. As Susan D. Block, MD and J. Andrew Billings, MD, "Learning from the Dying", *New England Journal of Medicine* (2005):353:1313-1315, accessed December 8, 2012, doi: 10.1056/ NEJMp048171, point out: "Students learn to elicit and value the patient's perspective and come to understand that each person's approach to dealing with illness is unique—a fundamental tenet of a patient-centered approach to doctoring." This training has value for upcoming physicians.

One 2007 graduate, Mauro Zappaterra, took the course because, as he said, "I didn't want to be the kind of physician who keeps his distance in order to keep his professionalism. The course gave me a template for how to talk about intimate things with patients and gave me permission to do it."

Throughout their years of training, students and physicians need to have opportunities to learn how to address death, dying, and the human experience of medical practice.

TOPICS IN THE END-OF-LIFE CURRICULUM

IF A PHYSICIAN is truly going to serve his or her patients, the doctor needs to be aware of what the German poet Rainer Maria Rilke calls the "the great death" for which a man prepares himself rather than the "little death" for which he is unprepared.

Medical schools must realize the importance of addressing spirituality as part of patient care as well as the doctors' own well-being.

Dr. M. Scott Peck, in his work *Denial of the Soul: Spiritual and Medical Perspectives on Euthanasia and Mortality*, suggests a course of training for medical professionals that includes:

- The concept of mortality and what it means to be mortal would be discussed.

- How death is denied in general in our society, and the Kübler Ross stages in particular, would be studied.
- Among other books, he would recommend reading Joseph Sharp's book *Living Our Dying: A Way to the Sacred in Everyday Life.*
- There would be a discussion of the afterlife and various belief systems about it.
- Students would explore various religions, including those that believe in karma and reincarnation.
- Discussion and exploration about ideas about the soul would occur.
- Considerable time would be spent on the ego and its involvement with the practice of medicine.
- Secular as well as religious ideas about meaning would be explored.
- There would be time for various ethical theories, with emphasis on ideal observer theory.
- There would be an exploration about distinctions between natural and human evil and how a supposedly loving God might permit these painful things.
- The euthanasia debate in all its ramifications would be included.

Dr. Ira Byock is the director of palliative medicine at Dartmouth Medical School as well as a faculty physician at this large teaching hospital. In his book *The Best Care Possible,* Dr. Byock states that our upcoming physicians are not as prepared as they should be in their training for treating and dealing with seriously ill and dying patients and their families. Dr. Byock sees that medical schools are underemphasizing topics and skills related to terminal conditions. Students are given no training on how to deliver the news that cancer has progressed or tell family members that a loved one has died. Topics such as how to introduce hospice care to a patient or how to employ CPR in a way that people can understand are not reviewed. Interns and residents often have only one lecture, if even, on pain management or on the ethics of stopping life-prolonging treatment plans. Residents are therefore left feeling incompetent in the area of allowing for a natural death, how to treat cancer pain, or how to encourage advance directives. Yet, most of these physicians will practice in the areas of family medicine, cardiology, neurology, internal medicine, oncology, infectious disease, critical care, general and oncology surgery, and other areas where a large portion of patients they see will be the dying elderly. These specialty doctors will, in fact, be providing to their patients end-of-life care. Should there not be adequate training for our doctors and nurses on this very subject?

Dr. Byock asks his third-year medical students to "think about the hours of coursework you have had on embryology, reproductive medicine, prenatal care, labor and delivery, and neonatal care, and about four- to six-week rotations in obstetrics and pediatrics that are required in this third year. Now, consider how many hours of required classes and clinical rotation are devoted to topics related to dying, caregiving, and grief? In this regard, as in most medical schools, our curriculum seems well suited to the 1940s and '50s, when most doctors delivered babies and routinely took care of infants." Yet, only about 50 percent of the American population will have children, and 100 percent will die.

It is time to change how our doctors and nurses are trained in this important area of death and dying. While it is valuable to have a course during their training, physicians also need learning opportunities and practice to address death, dying, and the human experience of medical practice. The continuing medical education programs can help these professions and their patients by offering expanded training in palliative care, as well as by making available faculty members who, at all stages of medical training, can teach these skills based on their own training and experiences.

As palliative care specialist Dr. Melissa Schepp states,

I think that if I had my, 'magic wand,' I would make it so that every caregiver knew a little bit about the basics of palliative care. Basically, that comfort is paramount, regardless of whether you are going for a cure or not. We need to pay more attention not just to pain management but good pain management.

I don't know what your destiny will be, but one thing I do know: the only ones among you who will be really happy are those who have sought and found how to serve.
~ Albert Schweitzer

CHAPTER FOURTEEN
The Future of End-of-Life Care

THE BABY BOOMER generation is taking note of how and in what ways their parents are dying. In the next years, the number of people who will face end-of-life choices will be incredible, and many of those will opt for hospice care. Like everything else this generation has done, this, too, will be done in a big way. Their choices about the care they will receive will have a profound effect on what becomes available for future generations.

The caregivers who were interviewed for this book say they are in conversations on a regular basis with the children of the patients they currently treat. These "children" are typically in their forties to their sixties. They have seen their grandparents—and now their mothers, fathers, aunts, and uncles—make their transition into the next life, and they are making decisions on how they want to orchestrate that experience for themselves. They often speak about themselves and say, "I want to age in place; I want to stay home. What do I have to do so I can age in place?" And that is becoming more prevalent. They want their deaths on their own terms as much as possible. They want to take ownership of their destiny and not leave it up to someone else. They want to be a part of the decision-making process. They want to be comfortable, with good palliative care and exercise the option of a good death. And they have already put it in writing.

HOSPICE IS BIG BUSINESS

IN A STUDY by Joshua E. Perry and Robert C. Stone, "In the Business of Dying: Questioning the Commercialization of Hospice," *Journal of Law, Medicine & Ethics*, 39: 224-234m diuL10,1111.h,1748-720/x,2011,0059,x, hospice care has evolved into "a multimillion dollar industry where the surviving nonprofits compete with for-profit providers, often publicly traded, managed by M.B.A.-trained executives, and governed by corporate boards."

According to the National Hospice and Palliative Care Organizaiton, *NHPCO Facts and Figures Hospice Care in America* (Alexandria), 2010, 9, there are almost five thousand hospices in the United States. As of 2009, 47 percent were for profit and 49 percent were nonprofit. The remaining 4 percent are government owned, such as veterans' hospices. The trend at this time appears to be the creation of more for-profit hospices, since their number has dramatically increased over the years. In fact, the number of for-profit hospices doubled between 2000 and 2007.

A *USA Today* article in 2011 pointed out that "From 2005 through 2009, Medicare spending on hospice care rose 70% to $4.31 billion, according to Medicare records." What will happen to those numbers as the baby boomers age and die? With that much money at stake, the door is opened for the further expansion of for-profit hospices.

However, hospice care is government regulated and, in many cases, paid for. At this writing, most believe the coming changes in the health-care industry will and must impact end-of-life care. Time will tell how that unfolds.

FOR-PROFIT HOSPICE VERSUS NONPROFIT HOSPICE

THE DIFFERENCE BETWEEN these two types of hospice is the business model. They both depend on government and insurance reimbursement to keep their doors open. While they are both cognizant of the bottom line, A for-profit hospice has owners and stockholders who are expecting a return on their money. A nonprofit hospice has a board of directors and must do fundraising to raise additional operating capital.

The demands of care often outweigh the per diem Medicare reimburses. Regardless of orientation, hospices are reimbursed the same. Nonprofits are able to fund raise and help support that. In hospice, the longer length of stay helps balance the more-expensive patients only in hospice for a short period of time. The most expensive time in hospice care is at the beginning and at the end of care. The patient who is in hospice for two weeks or less is an expensive client. Most of the high-intensity care takes place during the first two weeks of hospice care and the last two weeks of hospice care. These four weeks comprise the time when more nursing visits are needed and more medications are involved. Hospices must balance that expensive time by having patients who are on the service for months, allowing them to bill for that longer time period, which requires less attention and, therefore, helps them keep their bottom line in balance.

In addition, one way to make a greater profit is with volume; volume brings more profit. However, on the flip side is the choice to decrease services, so instead of having access to the services of a registered nurse twice a week, he or she might visit once a week and licensed practical nurses filling in with other visits.

Metta Johnson, who now runs her own consulting service, related her experience with one for-profit hospice. "Some of them even try not to supply all the supplies they are supposed to. I had a client on hospice, and she was dying of head and neck cancer, and the wounds had to be changed several times a day. Her husband did it, God bless him. They weren't providing him with gloves and gauze and all that. And, you know, I called because I know the regulations—Clyde and I were both nationally certified as administrators—and got them to provide the needed supplies."

She went on. "There is a profit to be made in hospice, but I think that the percentage of profit in that was our parting of the ways. We knew from being nationally certified care managers—certified hospice administrators—and talking to these people all over the United States that you can make about a 15 percent profit margin and provide good care. I think when you start looking for 35 percent and you are traded on the NY stock exchange, then it gets back to that one amount that you get for this patient and making the decision of how many ways are you going to divide it up."

The patient whose condition stabilizes somewhat and who needs less-intensive care for a longer period of time is a much more cost-effective client for the hospice. Between the two models, it is more likely the nonprofit will take the person who has very little or no monetary resources, no matter what their end-of-life care needs are. On the other hand, the for-profit hospice has a tendency to seek out those patients who require long-term care but do not have intensive and/or expensive medical needs.

A 2005 study in the *Journal of Palliative Medicine* found that large hospices owned by publicly traded companies generate profit margins nine times higher than those of large nonprofits. Michael J. McCue and Jon M. Thomson, "Operational and Financial Performance of Publicly Traded Hospice Companies", *Journal of Palliative Medicine* (2005):119-1206, doi:10.1089/jpm.2005.8.1196, "These cost savings and profit margins appear to flow primarily from business decisions relating to selective recruitment of a longer-term, increasingly non-cancerous, population of Medicare patients and the payment of lower salaries and benefits to less-skilled staff."

There are other issues to consider as well. There are ethical questions, such as the role of profit and its becoming the motivating factor for what your business does. For instance, do you keep a patient alive with artificial means—with nutrition when they no longer have an appetite, for example—and you're just promoting the growth of the cancer instead of letting nature take its course? Are you keeping them in a nursing home or hospice longer so that you can get the billing and make money? Will that be the trend?

On the other hand, why shouldn't hospice be a viable for-profit enterprise? It employs skilled people doing what they love to do, and offers myriad services to the patient (sometimes complementary services unavailable at a nonprofit). Why wouldn't a trained medical professional with good business sense, or even a large conglomerate, not want to become part of building a business with something to sell, with the knowledge that the business they built made a difference for the employees and the people they served?

While those who work in hospice are dedicated individuals who, for the most part, are called to the work they do, the main difference between profit and nonprofit is the bottom line. The for-profit hospice is first and foremost a business that must report to its owners and/or stockholders, and its purpose is to make money. However, that may or may not have anything to do with the care that is available. It is important to know who owns the hospice, but do not assume for profit is any better or worse than nonprofit. In any field of business, there are the good and the bad, and hospice is not different. There are ethical nonprofit corporations and ethical for-profit corporations just as there are unethical nonprofit or for-profit hospice corporations. The goals of any good hospice are the same—to provide high-quality care to the patient through employees who are highly trained and operate by offering heart-centered service.

When it comes to placing family members in hospice care, experts say, it's critical for families to ask questions to help make more-informed decisions. However, expect to see more marketing, including advertising, to get people to choose a particular hospice. For-profit hospices create significant marketing line items in their budgets in order to attract more people. Nonprofit hospices tend to have minimal or no marketing budgets, instead allocating their money for personnel and money for fund-raising efforts and market through those venues. Because of the competitive nature of all business, strategies for attracting clients are changing. Some of these can be very unsavory. Dawna White, a hospice nurse who writes the blog *allabouthospice.org,* says, "It's not the patient who's getting the hard sell; it's the hospitals and the doctors. If you ask your doctor for advice regarding hospice and are advised to use a specific hospice rather than offering a list of options, be sure to ask why."

Personal recommendations and your own feelings when visiting the hospice are the most important things to consider. Picking the wrong hospice can have disastrous effects in terms of your loved one's care. Do your own due diligence. When visiting the place you are considering, talk to the available staff. Look around you. How clean is it? How do patients look? What is the ambiance?

In addition, you need to be knowledgeable about the services you are entitled to receive. Be assertive in advocating for the needs of your loved one and your family. Be involved in the decision making that occurs.

Whether a hospice is for profit or nonprofit, it must be effectively managed with a close eye on the bottom line. It is up to the client, the patient and the family, to find the best option that is in alignment with their needs. As we move forward in time, this is going to become more and more necessary.

Choosing a Hospice

THERE IS NO shortage of dying patients. Rather than relying on marketing, advertising, or sales to obtain patients, wouldn't it be great if a facility's reputation preceded them and that was what invited a prospective patient to consider a particular hospice care organization?

Things to Take into Account when a Choosing Hospice

- Contact the National Hospice and Palliative Care Organization or the Hospice and Palliative Nurses Association to see what you can find out about a hospice.
- Find out how Medicare benefits work when someone is in hospice.
- You may also wish to get referrals from friends and hospital or nursing facility nurses. They are the front line in dealing with families and hospice care and often have very good information.
- Is the hospice for profit or nonprofit? Who owns it, and how is it run? Do they expect you to make a donation? Do they have any religious restrictions on the people it accepts?
- If considering an inpatient facility, be aware of, for lack of a better term, the "energy" you feel when you are there. Sometimes this can come in terms of visual cues—how well the facility maintained, how clean it is, and so on. Sometimes you just get a sense of peace or of "coming home" when you enter one of these facilities. Find out

what kind of accommodations are available for visitors. Can people stay overnight? Is there a playground or place for children? Are pets allowed?

- When talking with the representative of the hospice, find out what services the hospice offers. See if you can talk to family members of patients who have gone through the program. Ask about their experience with the services.

- Ask what happens after a patient is finished with the care at the hospice. What grief support do they provide or offer?

Families should talk with several hospice organizations and not sign anything until they have had time to think about it.

ALTERNATIVE PROGRAMS/CHOICES

PERHAPS YOUR LOVED one has a terminal illness, but the diagnosis is not sufficient to qualify for hospice. But he or she needs help on a hospice level. What do you do? Many people fall into this category, and there is a need to serve this demographic.

A new type of organization is becoming available throughout the country. They are called AIM programs—advanced illness management programs. Like hospice, these programs offer social support, case management, and nursing services. They are primarily home based and done in coordination with a patient's medical team. Some private insurance will pay for this service, however, at this time, Medicare and Medicaid does not.

Oftentimes AIM programs are offered in conjunction with cancer centers, and you may wish to investigate that option if there is a cancer center in your area. Other AIM programs are designed to help those coping with other advanced illness, such as stage 4 COPD, Parkinson's, or heart failure.

AIM programs are similar to hospice programs in many ways. However, they do not require a six-month prognosis as a prerequisite to enrollment which is the protocol hospices follow due to Medicare requirements. AIM programs usually allow the patient to continue active medical treatments when there is a late-stage illness.

IN THE FUTURE

MOST WHO CONTRIBUTED to this book felt end-of-life care of the future will grow from where it is today. It will include more of the mind, body, and spirit connection and expand into avenues of complementary care that will give comfort on an individual basis.

What if inpatient units were all beautiful, single rooms with an extra bed for overnight guests? They look out over courtyards, where children could play or guests and visitors could go and sit and talk. What if there was a hospice that included whatever the patient wanted or was available to be called on to let the patient experience music, art, or massage? How wonderful would it be if other modalities were available, such as chiropractic, Healing Touch, Reiki, energy work, chakra alignment, or acupuncture?

Currently, few of those things are either Medicare approved for payment or covered under private insurance. Therefore, either the hospice provides them and raises funds for it, or if the hospice is for profit, finds a way to pay for those services out of its profits. In a way, this is already governmentally set up, as payment is approved for the doctor, the nurse, the chaplain, and the social worker. But the massage therapist or musicians are not covered. Nor is there any approved avenue to make sure there is a way to take care of the dying person's pets; that's where volunteers come in right now. But the experience of death could be expanded to include a wide range of comfort care.

What if such a positive environment were created that patients knew they could feel like their hand was being held every step of the way, and they would never be alone in the walk they were taking. What if patients knew such a place existed before they needed it?

CONCLUSION

THERE WILL ALWAYS be people who have the heart for hospice. Regardless of whether they work in a for-profit or a nonprofit organization, there will always be those called to serve from the heart space those who need them at the end of life.

Ruth Donnellan, a massage therapist nurse, is able to do what she loves because the philosophy of where she works believes the needs, comfort, and care of the patient are primary—even if it includes the complementary care she offers, and it is taken out of the profit margin of the hospice. As she says, "I just have more faith in hospice than any other type of health care."

Afterword

No MATTER WHICH side of the current health-care reform debate you are on, most of us would like to see the physician acting in the best interest of the patient. A significant percentage of our current health-care costs (no one can even guess how much money is involved here) goes down the "defensive medicine" drain. Industry profits are set aside in the form of insurance premiums for individual or group physicians, other practitioners, and hospitals so that a patient who suffers injuries due to mistakes can be compensated.

In recent years, these malpractice premiums have been dropping due to widespread "cover your ass" behavior on the part of practitioners. Reckless and dangerous practices have disappeared, and overall care is better, but there has been a hidden price tag. Today we physicians are overcautious, inhibited, and afraid to trust our intuition. It is no fun to care for someone you view as a potential lawsuit, and physicians with their "shields up" order too many lab tests, X-rays, and consultations; they overutilize hospital services. Many patients with straightforward problems could be better served at the cost of one managed defensively. Our system has been absorbing these extra costs, but we all pay for them with higher premiums.

An alternative method for injured parties is to receive compensation, which eliminates the need to pay one-third of the settlement to the plaintiff's lawyer. Imagine a managed care plan that provides high-quality care at such a low price that members are willing to waive their right to bring a civil suit against the plan in favor of submitting grievances to an arbitration panel or administrative law judges, such as those hearing workers' compensation cases now. Each party could still have representation by a knowledgeable lawyer, as now, but these advocates would be paid hourly, not on a contingency basis.

The slow court system would be bypassed, justice would be swift, and the lessons learned in each case could help fine-tune the system almost immediately. More money would go directly to the deserving injured party, but despite this, overall costs would drop, as defensive medical care becomes a distant, bad memory. In order to study the feasibility of such a plan, new legislation would probably be needed, and adequate safeguards would have to be in place to protect the participants who voluntarily agree to waive or, perhaps, defer their constitutional right to a jury trial. In recent years, the federal government has encouraged competition and innovation by asking medical centers to submit ideas about how to build a better mousetrap. I would love to see variations of this idea put into practice and studied, and I would love to work for the managed care plan that rendered defensive medicine obsolete.

SETTING OUR SOCIAL PRIORITIES

As THE BABY boomers in our society reach retirement age, there will be more disease to diagnose and treat, and we will be forced to devote more resources to medical care. In the last few years, when medical spending approached 12 percent of the gross national product (GNP), there was a scream of protest from business and government leaders, and we got serious about medical cost-cutting. It is inevitable that spending for national defense worldwide will continue to decrease, and the savings will flow toward the more technical and expensive medical care of the future. Indeed, in a world beyond war, what could have a higher priority than our health? We have already made a commitment to offer basic medical care to our elderly (Medicare) and poor (Medicaid), and we are looking for ways to keep the working poor from falling through the cracks in our social net. A majority seem to favor continuing to expect employers to provide health insurance as a benefit to employees. We are all wary of switching to a government-dominated, single-payer system because of the problems encountered in countries where it has been tried and our basic belief that the government is too inefficient to manage something so complex as health care. The insurance company will continue to have a role, spreading risk and acting as a watchdog, although in my most idealistic, wild dream, this function is eliminated by a physician group capable of policing itself and delivering high-quality care in a cost-effective and compassionate manner.

THE MANAGED CARE PLAN OF THE NEXT CENTURY

IN OUR SOCIETY, we have powerful assets with which to build the ideal health-care system. We have a health-conscious and intelligent general population, an information system with radio, television, and the World Wide Web linking us all together more closely than we could have imagined just a few decades ago. We have health-care professionals who are well motivated, well informed, and who care for the well-being of their patients. Our hospitals spend profits on new equipment and are staffed by great nurses and other caregivers. Research continues as a matter of course, and new and better treatments are incorporated into our care plans rapidly. Our home-care capability is reaching its potential, and hospice care is more readily available to everyone. Many people utilize alternative or complementary practices, and the medical establishment is finding ways to find out which of these work and expand their use.

I predict that the next generations of managed-care plans will be able to offer excellent care at an affordable price by offering premium discounts for not smoking, being fit, maintaining an ideal weight, and so on. Preventive care will be the highest priority service, not just a window dressing, as now. Alternative treatments that work will be studied and incorporated into care plans. There will be no roadblocks to access to specialty care, and all serious illnesses will be managed by specialists. Advanced directives will be mandatory and honored scrupulously. Anyone with a limited prognosis will have early access to competent hospice care well before his or her last few days or weeks.

Futile care will not be offered as covered benefit, and any patient or family demanding aggressive care of this nature must "pay as you go" to have it continued. The psychospiritual costs of futile care for the patient, family, hospital staff, chaplains, and physicians are enormous. Not to mention the cost of squandered resources. Physicians will enjoy an excellent salary and benefit package, unfettered opportunity for research, good on call coverage, meeting allowances, paid malpractice premiums, and the hassle of running a business off their backs. The ideal managed-care system can be a win-win proposition for us all.

Robert Cowgill, MD
September 2004

Appendix I

The Dying Person's Bill of Rights

THIS BILL OF rights was created at the workshop "The Terminally Ill Patient and Helping Person," in Lansing, Michigan, sponsored by the SW Michigan Inservice Education Council and conducted by Amelia J. Barbus, associate professor of nursing, Wayne State University, Detroit. It is used extensively on various hospice-oriented Websites and was also featured in one of Ann Landers's columns.

- I have the right to be treated as a living human being until I die.
- I have the right to maintain a sense of hopefulness, however variable its focus may be.
- I have the right to be cared for by those who can maintain a sense of hopefulness, however variable this might be.
- I have the right to express my feelings and emotions about my approaching death in my own way.
- I have the right to participate in decisions concerning my illness.

- I have the right to expect continuing medical and nursing attention, even though "cure" goals must be changed to "comfort" goals.
- I have the right not to die alone.
- I have the right to be free of pain.
- I have the right to have any questions answered honestly.
- I have the right not to be deceived.
- I have the right to have help from and for my family in accepting my death.
- I have the right to die in peace and dignity.
- I have the right to retain my individuality and not be judged for my decisions which may be contrary to the beliefs of others.
- I have the right to discuss and enlarge my religious and/or spiritual experiences regardless of what they mean to others.
- I have the right to expect that the sanctity of the human body will be respected after death.
- I have the right to be cared for by caring, sensitive, knowledgeable people who will attempt to understand my needs and will be able to gain some satisfaction in helping me face death.

Appendix II

Resources

The resources below are provided for the benefit and information of the readers. The authors are not aligned with nor promote any of those listed.

Books

Abrahm, Janet, *A Physician's Guide to Pain and Symptom Management in Cancer Patients*, Baltimore: Johns Hopkins University Press, 2005.

Alexander, Eban, *Proof of Heaven*, New York: Simon & Schuster, 2012.

Byock, Ira, *Dying Well: The Prospect for Growth at the End of Life*, New York: Riverhead Books, 1997.

Byock, Ira, *The Best Care Possible: A Physician's Quest to Transform Care through the End of Life*, New York: Penguin, 2012.

Callanan, Maggie, *Final Journeys: A Practical Guide for Bringing Care and Comfort at the End of Life,* New York: Bantam Books, 2009.

Callanan, Maggie, and Patricia Kelley, *Final Gifts: Understanding the Special Awareness, Needs, and Communications of the Dying,* New York: Bantam Books, 1997.

Davies, Douglas James, *A Brief History of Death (Blackwell Brief Histories of Religion),* Malden, MA: Blackwell Publishing, 2005.

Duda, Deborah, *Coming Home: A Practical and Compassionate Guide to Caring for a Dying Loved One,* Austin, TX: Synergy Books, 2010.

Feldman, David B., and Andrew Lasher Jr, *The End-of-Life Handbook: A Compassionate Guide to Connecting with and Caring for a Dying Loved One,* Oakland: New Harbinger Publications, 2007.

Jones, Phillip, *Light on Death: The Spiritual Art of Dying,* San Rafael, CA: Mandala Publishing, 2007.

Kessler, David, *The Needs of the Dying: A Guide for Bringing Hope, Comfort, and Love to Life's Final Chapter,* New York: HarperCollins Publishers, 2007.

Kübler-Ross, Elisabeth, *On Death and Dying,* New York: Touchstone, 1997.

Kuhl, David, *What Dying People Want: Practical Wisdom for the End of Life,* New York: Public Affairs, 2002.

Lief, Judith, *Making Friends with Death: A Buddhist Guide to Encountering Mortality,* Boston: Shambhalah Publications, Inc., 2001.

Long, Jeffrey, with Paul Perry, *Evidence of the Afterlife: The Science of Near-Death Experiences,* NewYork: HarperOne, 2010.

Lynn, Joanne, Janice Lynch Schuster, and Joan Harrold, *Handbook for Mortals: Guidance for People Facing Serious Illness,* New York: Oxford University Press, 2011.

Madden, Kristine, *Shamanic Guide to Death and Dying,* New York: Spilled Candy Publications, 2005.

Moody, Raymond, *Life after Life,* San Francisco: Harper Collins, 1975.

Moody, Raymond, *Reflections on Life after Life,* New York: Bantam Books, 1983.

Moody, Raymond, *The Light Beyond,* New York: Bantam Books, 1988.

Moody, Raymond, *Coming Back: A Psychiatrist Explores Past Life Journeys,* New York: Bantam Books, 1991.

Moody, Raymond, *The Last Laugh: A New Philosophy of Near Death Experiences, Apparitions, and the Paranormal,* Charlottesville, VA: Hampton Roads, 1999.

Moody, Raymond, and Deanne Arcangel, *Life after Loss: Conquering Grief and Finding Hope,* New York: Harper Collins, 2001.

Moody, Raymond, and Paul Perry, *Reunions: Visionary Encounters with Departed Loved Ones,* New York: Ballantine Books, 1993.

Moody, Raymond, and Paul Perry, *Glimpses of Eternity,* New York: Guideposts, 2010.

Moody, Raymond, and Paul Perry, *Paranormal: My Life in Pursuit of the Afterlife,* New York: HarperOne, 2012.

Musgrave, Beverly A., and McGettigan, Neil, *Spiritual and Psychological Aspects of Illness: Dealing with Sickness, Loss, Dying, and Death,* Mahwah, NJ: Paulist Press, 2010.

Neal, Mary C., *To Heaven and Back: A Doctor's Extraordinary Account of Her Death, Heaven, Angels, and Life Again: A True Story,* Colorado Springs: Waterbrook Press, 2012.

Nuland, Sherwin B., *How We Die: Reflections of Life's Final Chapter,* New York: First Vintage Books, 1994.

Peck, M. Scott, *Denial of the Soul: Spiritual and Medical Perspectives on Euthanasia and Mortality,* New York: Harmony Books, 1997.

Quill, Timothy E., *Death and Dignity: Making Choices and Taking Charge,* New York: Norton & Company, 1993.

Quill, Timothy E., *A Midwife through the Dying Process: Stories of Healing and Hard Choices at the End of Life,* Baltimore: Johns Hopkins University Press, 1996.

Quill, Timothy E., *Caring for Patients at the End of Life: Facing an Uncertain Future Together,* New York: Oxford University Press, 2001.

Quill, Timothy E., and Margaret P. Battin, *Physician-Assisted Dying: The Case for Palliative Care and Patient Choice,* 2004.

Remen, Rachel Naomi, *My Grandfather's Blessings: Stories of Strength, Refuge and Belonging,* New York: The Berkley Publishing Group, 2001.

Remen, Rachel Naomi, *Kitchen Table Wisdom: Stories that Heal,* New York: The Berkley Publishing Group, 2006

Rinpoche, Sogyal, *The Tibetan Book of Living and Dying,* San Francisco: Harper Collins, 1994.

Rosen, Steven J., *Ultimate Journey: Death and Dying in the World's Major Religions,* Westport, CT: Praeger Publishers, 2008.

Sanders, Mary Anne, *Nearing Death Awareness: A Guide to the Language, Visions and Dreams of the Dying,* Philadelphia and London: Jessica Kingsley Publishers, 2007.

Sharp, Joseph, *Living Our Dying: A Way to the Sacred in Everyday Life,* New York: Hyperion Books, 1997.

Shavelson, Lonny, *A Chosen Death: The Dying Confront Assisted Suicide,* Berkeley: University of California Press, 1998.

Smith, Jane Idelman, and Yvonne Yazbeck Haddad, *The Islamic Understanding of Death and Resurrection,* New York: Oxford University Press, 2002.

Snyder, Lois, and Timothy E. Quill, *Physician's Guide to End-of-Life Care,* Philadelphia: American College of Physicians-American Society of Internal Medicine, 2001.

Stanworth, Rachel, *Recognizing Spiritual Needs in People Who Are Dying,* New York: Oxford University Press, 2004.

Wooten-Green, Ronald, and Joseph M. Champlin, *When the Dying Speak: How to Listen to and Learn from Those Facing Death,* Chicago: Loyola Press, 2001.

Blogs

Please note: descriptions of blogs come from the blogs themselves.

Caring.com
www.caring.com
Founded in 2007, Caring.com is the leading online destination for those seeking information and support as they care for aging parents, spouses, and other loved ones. Our mission: to help the helpers. We equip family caregivers to make better decisions, save time and money, and feel less alone -- and less stressed -- as they face the many challenges of caregiving.

There are blogs on different topics related to caregiving and end of life issues.

Hospice and Caregiving Blog
http://blog.hospicefoundation.org/

The Hospice and Caregiving Blog is maintained by the Hospice Foundation of America (HFA). The blog was started in September 2007 to share stories and articles relating to hospice and palliative care, end-of-life experiences, caregiving, and grief and bereavement. Along with the articles developed by our regular contributors, the Hospice and Caregiving Blog offers updates on general media coverage of these topics, as well as profiles of professionals involved in related fields.
medicalfutility.blogspot.com

GeriPal—A Geriatrics and Palliative Care Blog
www.geripal.org

The objectives are (1) to create an online community of interdisciplinary providers interested in geriatrics or palliative care; (2) to provide an open forum for the exchange of ideas and disruptive commentary that changes clinical practice and health-care policy; and (3) to change the world.

Organizations/Websites

All descriptions are from the sites themselves.

American Hospice Foundation
www.americanhospice.org

The foundation's goal is to improve access to quality hospice care through public education, professional training, and advocacy on behalf of consumers.

Americans for Better Care of the Dying
www.abcd-caring.org
Founded in 1997, Americans for Better Care of the Dying (ABCD) is dedicated to ensuring all Americans can count on good end-of-life care. Our goals are to
- Build momentum for reform
- Explore new methods and systems for delivering care
- Shape public policy through evidence-based understanding

Accomplishment of these goals is done by focusing efforts on fundamental reforms, such as improved pain management, better financial reimbursement systems, enhanced continuity of care, support for family caregivers, and changes in public policy.

"The End of Life: Exploring Death in America"
www.npr.org/programs/death/
This is the Website for the NPR program, "The End of Life: Exploring Death in America."

Home Hospice Foundation of America
www.hospicefoundation.org
HFA's Hospice Information Center offers testimonials, educational programs, videos, and downloadable fact sheets about end-of-life care, available at no cost

Hospice Patients Alliance
www.hospicepatients.org

The Hospice Patients Alliance was formed in August of 1998 as a nonprofit charitable organization and is a 501(c)(3) corporation serving the general public throughout the United States. We were formed by experienced hospice staff and other health care professionals who saw that hospices were not always complying with the standards of care, and in fact, were in some cases, violating the rights of patients and families and exploiting them for financial gain, or not providing adequate care to control pain or other distressing symptoms during the end of life period.

IPCRC.net, the International Palliative Care Resource Center
www.ipcrc.net
The IPCRC is dedicated to
- Making palliative care resources accessible for health-care professionals
- Building palliative care capacity worldwide
- Providing a dynamic and constantly expanding Website

LIFE before Death
www.lifebeforedeath.com/movie/index.shtml
LIFE before Death is a documentary project comprising a feature film, a one-hour television program, and fifty short films about the global crisis in untreated pain and the dramatic, life-changing affect palliative care services can deliver to patients and their families.

National Alliance for Caregivers
www.caregiving.org
Established in 1996, The National Alliance for Caregiving is a non-profit coalition of national organizations focusing on issues of family caregiving. Alliance members include grassroots

organizations, professional associations, service organizations, disease-specific organizations, a government agency, and corporations.

The National Association for Home Care & Hospice
www.nahc.org/
This is the site of the country's largest trade association representing the interests and concerns of home care agencies, hospices, and home care aide organizations.

National Hospice and Palliative Care Organization
www.nhpco.org/templates/1/homepage.cfm
The National Hospice and Palliative Care Organization (NHPCO) is the largest nonprofit membership organization representing hospice and palliative care programs and professionals in the United States. The organization is committed to improving end of life care and expanding access to hospice care with the goal of profoundly enhancing quality of life for people dying in America and their loved ones.

National Center for Complementary and Alternative Medicine
www.nccam.nih.gov
The National Center for Complementary and Alternative Medicine (NCCAM) is the federal government's lead agency for scientific research on the diverse medical and health-care systems, practices, and products that are not generally considered part of conventional medicine.

National Center for Complementary and Alternative Medicine
www.nccam.nih.gov
The National Center for Complementary and Alternative Medicine (NCCAM) is the federal government's lead agency

for scientific research on the diverse medical and health-care systems, practices, and products that are not generally considered part of conventional medicine.

National Healthcare Decisions Day

www.nhdd.org

The National Healthcare Decisions Day (NHDD) Initiative is a collaborative effort of national, state, and community organizations committed to ensuring all adults with decision-making capacity in the United States have the information and opportunity to communicate. NHDD exists to inspire, educate, and empower the public and providers about the importance of advance care planning

The Robert Wood Johnson Foundation

www.rwjf.org

The Robert Wood Johnson Foundation focuses on the pressing health and health-care issues facing our country. It is the nation's largest philanthropy devoted exclusively to improving the health and health care of all Americans. It works with a diverse group of organizations and individuals to identify solutions and achieve comprehensive, meaningful, and timely change. For more than thirty-five years, the foundation has brought experience, commitment, and a rigorous, balanced approach to the problems that affect the health and health care of those it serves. Helping Americans lead healthier lives and get the care they need, the foundation expects to make a difference in our lifetime.

The Twilight Brigade

www.thetwilightbrigade.com

The Twilight Brigade is one of the largest end-of-life care communities. It operates as an independent agency within VA hospitals and hospice care facilities across America.

The Twilight Brigade chair, Dannion Brinkley, and the approximately five thousand volunteers nationwide who make up The Twilight Brigade, are dedicated to being at the bedside of our nation's dying, especially veterans.

Hospice or Palliative Care

American Hospice Foundation
1-800-347-1413
www.americanhospice.org

National Hospice and Palliative Care Organization
1-800-658-8898
www.nhpco.org

Centers for Medicare & Medicaid Services
1-800-633-4227
www.medicare.gov

Visiting Nurse Associations of America
1-202-384-1420
www.vnaa.org

Department of Veterans Affairs
1-877-222-8387
www.va.org

Center to Advance Palliative Care
1-212-201-2670
www.getpalliativecare.org

The site provides clear, comprehensive palliative care information for people coping with serious, complex illness. Key components of the site include a Palliative Care Directory of Hospitals, a definition of palliative care, and a detailed description of what palliative care is and how it is different from hospice. It also provides an interactive questionnaire to assist people in determining whether palliative care is appropriate for them or their loved ones.

Children's Hospice International
http://www.chionline.org/
Through the efforts of Children's Hospice International most of the over three thousand hospices in the United States will now consider accepting children. Also, approximately 450 programs have children-specific hospice, palliative, or home-care services. Among the independent children's hospice homes are

- George Mark Children's Hospice, opened March 2004 in California
- Ryan House, opened March 2010 in Arizona
- Dr. Bob's Place, set to open in 2011 in Maryland
- Sarah House, in development in Ohio
- Connor's House, in development in Philadelphia
- Children's Lighthouse of Minnesota, in development in Minnesota
- Providence TrinityCare Hospice, serving Los Angeles and Orange counties in California

Advance Directives and Living Wills

American Bar Association
1-800-285-2221
www.abanet.org

Caring Connection (National Hospice and Palliative Care Organization)
1-800-658-8898
www.caringinfo.org

Medlineplus
www.medlineplus.gov
Click on "Advance Directives."

National Cancer Institute
800-422-6237
www.cancer.gov

Other Types of Complementary Care for Those at the End of Life

What follows is a list of organizations that offer comfort. Some are national; others are regional. It is not a complete list but includes those we came into contact with during our research.

The Sacred Dying Foundation
www.sacreddying.org
The Sacred Dying philosophy is concerned with bringing spirituality, through presence and ritual, into the physical act of dying. Sacred Dying facilitates the creation of a setting where death is experienced with honor, respect, and sacredness. This can be as simple as being present with a loved one or as complicated as transforming the vision of our entire society. It is a proven approach to providing spiritual aid to the dying and their loved ones.

It is part of the No One Dies Alone program and offers training.

Chalice of Repose Project
chaliceofrepose.org
Music-thanatology is a subspecialty of palliative medicine, and derives profound spiritual inspiration and meaning from the Benedictine Cluniac tradition of monastic medicine. In that light, every moment, person, condition, and event is one in which we can turn to greet, receive, and meet one another "in a new and living way."

Keep the Spirit of '45 Alive!
www.spiritof45.org
Keep the Spirit of '45 Alive! is a nonprofit, nonpartisan initiative to preserve the legacy of the men and women of the "Greatest Generation," so their example of courage, self-sacrifice, "can-do" attitude, and commitment to community can help inspire a renewal of national unity in America at a time when our country once again must come together to meet historic challenges.

The organization's goal is to establish an annual day of remembrance and national renewal to remind America of the values and accomplishments of the generation who endured the hard times of the Great Depression, fought to defeat the greatest tyranny in history, and then went on to rebuild their shattered world in an unprecedented effort to help assure a better future for both friend and former foe alike.

Happy Tails Pet Therapy
www.happytailspets.org
Just about every city has a pet therapy program that serves those who are seriously ill or dying. To find one in your area, Google pet therapy and your city. In the metro Atlanta area, for example, there is a wonderful organization called Happy Tails, which was founded by Atlanta veterinarian Carla Courtney. Happy Tails volunteers share the unconditional love of their pets with people

of all ages with physical, social, emotional, and cognitive needs at health-care facilities, social agencies, and special needs programs in the metro Atlanta community.

Bay Kids
www.baykids.org
Located in the San Francisco Bay area, BayKids empowers children facing serious medical challenges to express themselves through the art and magic of filmmaking. BayKids teaches digital filmmaking skills to hospitalized children. Through the program, children discover their own unique voice and experience the healing power of self-expression.

Near-Death Experiences

The International Association for Near-Death Studies (IANDS)
iands.org/home.html
IANDS promotes responsible, multidisciplinary exploration of near-death and similar experiences, their effects on people's lives, and their implications for beliefs about life, death, and human purpose.
In addition to this Website, IANDS publishes a peer-reviewed scholarly journal and a member newsletter, sponsors conferences and other programs, works with the media, and encourages the formation of regional discussion and support groups.

Eben Alexander, III, MD
www.lifebeyonddeath.net
A neurosurgeon who experienced a near-death experience.

Raymond A. Moody, MD
www.lifeafterlife.com
The official online presence of Dr. Raymond A. Moody.

About the Authors

ROBERT COWGILL, MD

HOSPICE PIONEER DR. Robert Cowgill adopted a holistic approach to helping his cancer patients. He became one of the first hospice medical directors in Atlanta. The hospice work he did in addition to his private surgical practice was his passion and his spiritual calling. He was involved before his death in trying to get established a newly emerging palliative care unit at the hospital he worked with in Atlanta. Dr. Cowgill served as a past president of a chapter of the American Cancer Society. For many years, he was actively involved as a facilitator for an ongoing cancer support group.

Although a Western trained surgeon, Dr. Cowgill had a decidedly Eastern philosophy toward spiritual matters. He incorporated into the healing process the importance of the mind and body connection and the spiritual/emotional aspect of medical care. He never touted this alone as the cure for medical problems but saw it as a complement to the total treatment plan. Dr. Cowgill was also open to the use of prayer if the patient wished for this. He did not care that his fellow physicians may not have approved of the unconventional methods he used with his patients; he did what he felt was the right thing to do for that patient's spirit and emotional well-being as well as his or her physical body.

Graduated from the University of Virginia School of Medicine, Dr. Cowgill received his internship in surgery at Emory University Affiliated Hospitals and his residency training in general surgery at Georgia Baptist Hospital in Atlanta, Georgia. In 1976, he was awarded a fellowship from the American Cancer Society in surgical oncology at Memorial Sloan-Kettering Cancer Center. He was clinical instructor in surgery at Cornell Medical School and the New York Hospital. He served as senior consultant in surgery at King Faisal Specialist Hospital in Saudi Arabia and in the US Army Medical Corps active duty. He was certified by the American Board of Surgery.

In 1978, Dr. Cowgill became the first medical director of Hospice Atlanta and remained involved in the field until his death in 2006. At that time, he was serving as medical director of VITAS Innovative Hospice Care, formerly Haven House Hospice, as well as maintaining a private surgical oncology practice.

CHRISTINE COWGILL, MS, CRC

AS AN ADVOCATE for those returning to the workforce after an injury, Christine Cowgill has spent her life in service to those in need. As a certified rehabilitation counselor, she has worked to provide medical and vocational case management services to insurance companies on workers' compensation files. Christine Cowgill is also a licensed life and health insurance agent.

Christine Cowgill is a graduate of Kendall College with a degree in human services. She received her graduate degree in rehabilitation counseling from Georgia State University.

She has a wide range of interests and gives of her time in her community pursuits. She has been a volunteer social action coordinator with a church community, organizing activities such as hunger and AIDS walks. In 1993, she was honored as an individual winner by the Atlanta Committee for Olympic Games for organizing, in conjunction with a Catholic church, the first Meals on Wheels route to persons with AIDS in Cobb County, Georgia.

Writing the book her husband started has been a service of love as well as a life-changing experience for her.

CPSIA information can be obtained at www.ICGtesting.com
Printed in the USA
LVOW060519120213

319632LV00001B/79/P